Final Steps: End-of-Life Care for Dementia

Laura Town and Karen Hoffman

Omega Press
Zionsville, IN 46077

ISBN: 978-1-943414-09-3

Production Credits:
Authors: Laura Town and Karen Hoffman
Publisher: Omega Press
Photos: All credited images used under license from Shutterstock.com

Social media connections:

Laura Town
Twitter: @laurawtown
LinkedIn: https://www.linkedin.com/in/lauratown

Karen Hoffman
LinkedIn: https://www.linkedin.com/in/karen-hoffman-91502b62/

Omega Press in the News

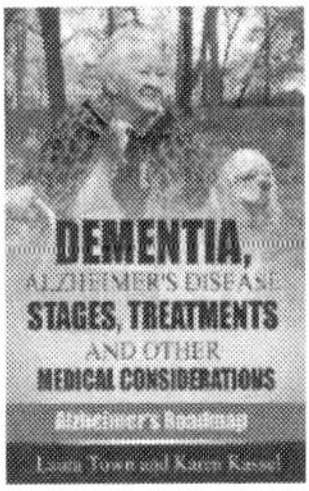

Dementia, Alzheimer's Disease Stages, Treatments, and Other Medical Considerations

- One of Book Authority's best books on dementia of all time
- One of Book Authority's best audiobooks on dementia of all time
- Audiobook recognized as a resource by the Alzheimer's Association
- Recommended by Dementia Insight
- Recommended by Alzheimer's Proof website
- Audiobook, ebook, and paperback available wherever books are sold

Long-Term Care Insurance, Power of Attorney, Wealth Management, and Other First Steps

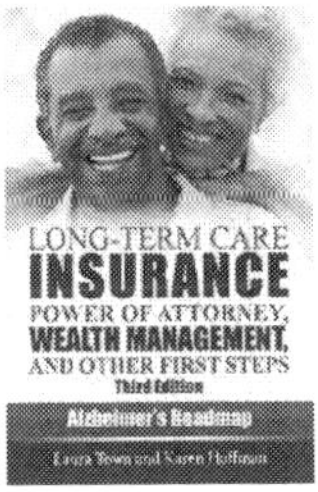

- One of Book Authority's best new insurance books to read in 2020
- Audiobook, ebook, and paperback available on Amazon

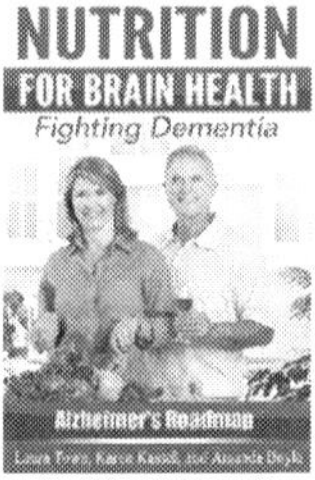

Nutrition for Brain Health: Fighting Dementia

- A Seniorlink (www.seniorlink.com) 50 Essential Read for Anyone Coping with Alzheimer's Disease
- Audiobook, ebook, and paperback available wherever books are sold

CONTENTS

Chapter 1: End-of-Life Symptoms

The final stage of Alzheimer's disease is often a mixture of heartbreak and relief for loved ones: Heartbreak because your loved one's mental and physical condition has deteriorated significantly, but relief that the struggle is almost over. This book will discuss what to expect at the end of your loved one's life, including physical and mental symptoms, the need for palliative care vs. hospice care, the grieving process, and practical matters related to funeral arrangements and your loved one's estate.

Just like the other stages of Alzheimer's disease, individuals with Alzheimer's disease display common symptoms related to the end of life. However, the way the symptoms exhibit themselves and when the symptoms appear may differ between individuals. Because the mind has stopped functioning normally, many basic bodily processes begin to shut down at the end of life. The inability to swallow affects your loved one's ability to take in nutrition and fluids and can lead to aspiration pneumonia. Similarly, the inability to move independently makes your loved one susceptible to pressure ulcers, which can also develop infections. In addition, individuals with Alzheimer's disease may not be able to tell you what is wrong, so you will need to watch for clues and try to address each issue as it arises. The following checklist provides a general overview of symptoms that indicate that the end of life may be near. It is important to remember that the end of life involves many of these symptoms being present simultaneously, so the appearance of any

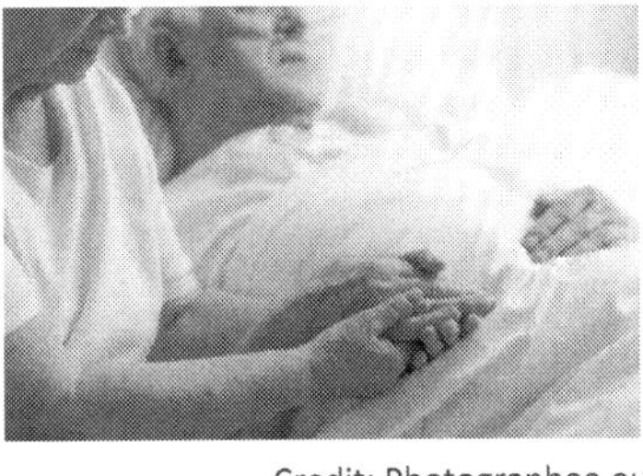

Credit: Photographee.eu

symptom in isolation (fatigue, for example, or low blood pressure) is not indicative of the approach of death. Instead, death is approaching when many of these symptoms appear together because of the collapse of the dying person's body functions.

Checklist: End-of-life symptoms

- ☐ Neurological symptoms
    - Agitation and aggression
    - Pain
    - Speech limited to a few words a day
    - Fatigue
    - Body jerking or seizures
    - Groaning or moaning
    - Increased sleeping
- ☐ Respiratory symptoms
    - Difficulty breathing
    - Apnea
    - Death rattle
- ☐ Cardiovascular symptoms
    - Low blood pressure
    - Poor circulation
    - Irregular pulse

- ☐ Integumentary (skin) symptoms
    - o Dry and fragile skin
    - o Cold hands, feet, and legs
    - o Mottled skin
    - o Pressure ulcers
    - o Poor temperature regulation
- ☐ Digestive symptoms
    - o Weight loss
    - o Loss of bowel control
- ☐ Musculoskeletal symptoms
    - o Unable to move independently
    - o Difficulty swallowing
    - o Difficulty controlling the head
- ☐ Urinary symptoms
    - o Loss of bladder control
    - o Inadequate urine production
- ☐ Immune symptoms
    - o Increased vulnerability to infections
- ☐ Diagnosis of another serious condition such as cancer or heart failure

The next several checklists examine specific end-of-life symptoms in greater detail. In considering these various symptoms, remember that the goal of care at this stage is relieving pain and distress. The point of care is to improve comfort and relieve suffering, not to cure the person. So where typically signs and symptoms are used to identify specific conditions to treat, with end-of-life signs and symptoms, the condition causing the signs and symptoms is less important to identify. Instead, focus on treating the signs and symptoms and providing palliative care and comfort to the individual.

Checklist: Agitation and aggression

- ☐ Agitation often indicates that the person is worried about something, which may cause sleeplessness or aggression.
- ☐ Aggression is when the person lashes out verbally or tries to hit or hurt someone.
- ☐ Agitation and aggression are often caused by an underlying condition:
    - Pain
    - Depression
    - Too little sleep
    - Constipation
    - Soiled diaper
    - Sudden changes
    - Too much noise
    - Being pushed to do something against the person's will (such as bathe or remember troubling events or people)

- Lack of contact with people
- Medication interactions

□ If you see signs of agitation or aggression, try to identify the underlying problem and deal with it before any problem behaviors start.

□ Sometimes, medication such as an antipsychotic may be necessary if the person is at risk of harming self or others.

□ Ways to cope with agitation or aggression:

- Speaking calmly and listening to what the person has to say
- Keeping a routine
- Building in quiet times during the day
- Surrounding the person with items they love
- Using gentle touches if your loved one allows them
- Reducing noise, clutter, and number of people in the room

Checklist: Pain

□ People with Alzheimer's disease often cannot tell you where they hurt or how bad the pain is.

□ Watch for signs of pain and treat pain early. It is easier to prevent pain then to reduce severe pain.

□ Signs of pain in people with Alzheimer's disease:

- Frequent position changes or restlessness

    - Having trouble sleeping
    - Increased agitation
    - Crying or moaning
    - Grimacing
    - Sweating

- ☐ Agitation may indicate that your loved one is in pain and cannot tell you.

- ☐ A refusal to eat may indicate tooth pain or other oral health issues.

- ☐ Some family members or physicians may not want to use narcotics or other strong or addictive pain medications because of their addictive properties. However, for individuals with Alzheimer's disease at the end of life, addiction is not a concern, so treatment should be sufficient to reduce the pain level.

- ☐ If the medication is not successful at relieving pain, speak to a doctor, nurse, or pain specialist.

- ☐ Some pain medications may cause side effects, such as constipation or dry mouth. Watch for these side effects and have a plan to manage them.

- ☐ One common side effect of narcotics/opioids prescribed for pain is respiratory depression (slow and shallow breathing). Individuals with Alzheimer's may have trouble breathing anyway, so you need to watch for this carefully.

- ☐ At the end of life, administration of doses of narcotics large enough to adequately manage pain may result in your loved one being semi-conscious or unconscious most of the time, potentially even until the time of death. Be prepared for this reality.

Checklist: Changes in breathing patterns

- ☐ Difficulty breathing (called dyspnea) is common at the end of life.
- ☐ Breathing problems may also include apnea (periods without breathing) or shallow breathing.
- ☐ Strategies to improve breathing:
    - Raising the head of the bed
    - Propping up the person with pillows
    - Opening a window or using a fan
    - Using a humidifier
- ☐ Individuals near death often have noisy breathing. This is called a death rattle. The death rattle occurs because excess secretions from the throat collect in the throat and cause a gurgling sound with each breath. You can reduce the death rattle by turning the person on one side.

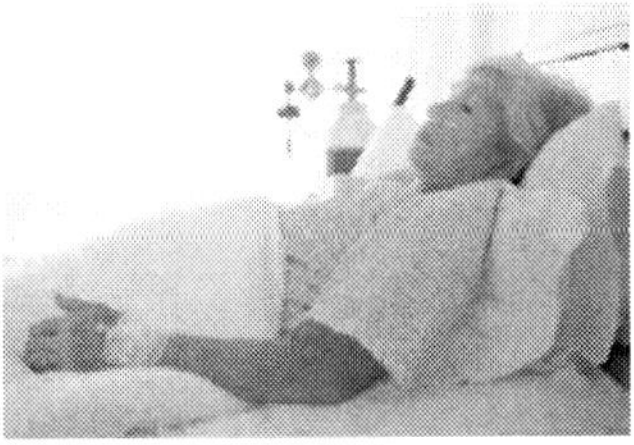

Credit: Akkalak Aiempradit

- ☐ Keep in mind that all noisy breathing is not a death rattle and is not usually upsetting to the person who is dying; it is usually more distressing for their loved ones.
- ☐ Cheyne-Stokes breathing occurs when the individual takes several breaths followed by a long

pause before regular breathing resumes. This pattern of breathing frequently occurs as individuals approach death.

Checklist: Cardiovascular problems

- ☐ At the end of life, the individual's blood pressure will drop below normal.
- ☐ Low blood pressure, dehydration, and inefficient heart pumping contribute to poor circulation.
- ☐ Signs of poor circulation include extremities that are cool to the touch and cyanosis (bluish color) of the lips and nails.
- ☐ To stimulate circulation, gently massage the hands and feet with lotion.
- ☐ Keeping the person warm (but not too warm) can also promote circulation to the hands and feet.
- ☐ Many individuals with Alzheimer's disease develop cardiovascular problems such as congestive heart failure at the end of life. In congestive heart failure, the heart can no longer pump effectively. This can be caused by a variety of reasons.
- ☐ Failure of the heart to pump effectively can lead to an irregular pulse.
- ☐ If the patient has an irregular pulse accompanied by agitation or restlessness, look for causes for this behavior such as pain or thirst.

Checklist: Skin problems

- ☐ As people age, their skin becomes drier and more fragile, increasing the risk for skin problems and infections.

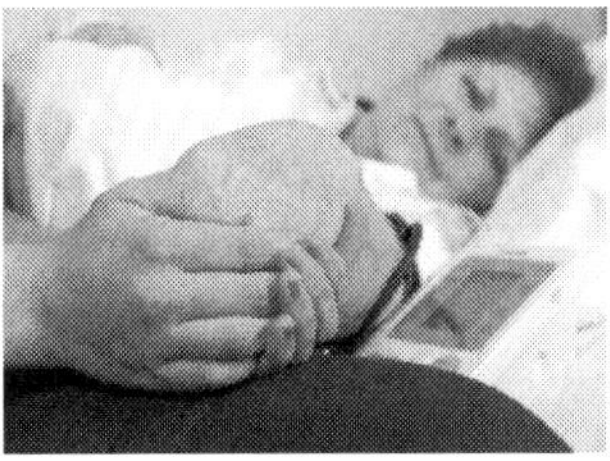

Credit: Ocskav Mark

- ☐ Near death, dryness of the lips and eyes is common. Use a lip balm or a damp cloth over the eyes to relieve dryness.

- ☐ Check your loved one's feet for cuts and other issues. Put lotion on his or her feet and cut or file toenails. If your loved one has sores on the feet, talk to a foot care doctor.

- ☐ Your loved one's skin may become mottled, which is means it has a blotchy, reddish marbling of the skin. It is not painful, and it usually occurs in the final week of life, typically beginning in the feet and traveling up the legs.

- ☐ Individuals with Alzheimer's disease who are at the end of life are often unable to move independently and are bed-bound or wheelchair-bound, so they are at higher risk for developing pressure ulcers.

- ☐ Pressure ulcers have four stages. They start at Stage 1 with redness at the pressure site and potential changes in sensation or temperature, and they end at Stage 4 with full-thickness loss of skin and exposure of muscle and bone.

- ☐ Common locations for pressure ulcers include the heels, hips, buttocks, shoulders, lower back, elbows, and back of the head.

- □ Pressure sores can be prevented by turning the person from side to side every 1-2 hours and by putting a foam pad under the area to reduce pressure. They can also be prevented by regularly helping your loved one with movement of the arms and legs.

- □ Individuals with Alzheimer's disease who are at the end of life may be sensitive to temperature extremes, but they may not be able to tell you if they are too hot or too cold.

- □ If your loved one is too hot, he or she might try to remove a blanket repeatedly. You can help by taking off the blanket and placing a cool cloth on the head.

- □ If your loved one is too cold, he or she might be hunched or shivering. Raise the heat and add another blanket to the person's covers. Avoid electric blankets that could burn the person's skin.

- □ Near the end of life, your loved one's hands, feet, arms, and legs may be cold to the touch.

Checklist: Digestive and eating problems

- □ Your loved one may become unaware of anything having to do with food, including meal times and choosing appropriate foods.

- □ Digestive problems at the end of life include nausea, vomiting, constipation, and loss of appetite. Speak to a doctor about what medications are available to treat digestive symptoms.

- □ Always make sure your loved one is sitting up and fully awake before eating. Your loved one should remain in an upright position for at least 20-30 minutes after the meal.

- For some individuals, eating may cause more discomfort. Therefore, do not try to force your loved one to eat.

- If your loved one is willing to eat, don't rush them. Allow them to take time to chew and swallow each bite.

- If your loved one is taking hours to eat a meal, consider that they have potentially forgotten how to eat or the purpose of eating. Patiently coax them to eat as much as possible.

- Individuals with Alzheimer's disease at the end of life often have trouble swallowing, so they may be unable to eat or drink on their own.

- If your loved one is still able to swallow but cannot feed themselves, you can help with feeding favorite foods in small amounts, choosing foods that are easy to chew and swallow, and choosing healthy, high-calorie foods.

- At the end of life, your loved one may stop eating and drinking altogether. This does not cause suffering for the individual.

- Individuals with Alzheimer's disease can easily become dehydrated because they forget to drink or because their thirst reflex is gone. Use ice chips to keep the person's mouth moist if they

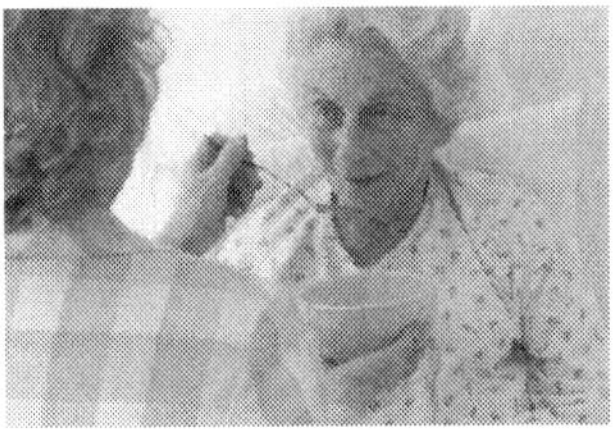

Credit: JPC-PROD

cannot swallow. Lip balm can also help keep the lips moistened.

- For oral health, use a Q-tip dipped in lemon water to swab the mouth. This keeps the mucous membranes moist and helps freshen the breath.

- Individuals with Alzheimer's disease often suffer from constipation, diarrhea, or bowel incontinence.

- Constipation involves a less-than-usual number of bowel movements. This can be a side effect of some medications or an effect of disease, diet, or decreased activity. Some over-the-counter medications can help with constipation, and changes in diet also help, such as drinking more liquids. Talk to a dietician about dietary interventions that are appropriate for your loved one.

- Diarrhea involves loose and watery bowel movements, which can contribute to dehydration. Over-the-counter medications can help. Keep the person with diarrhea hydrated with clear liquids. The person's rectum must also be kept clean with gentle washing with soap and water and the application of an ointment after each bowel movement.

- If your loved one is bed-bound and has difficulty controlling bowel movements, adult incontinence pads can be used. Incontinence pads should be changed frequently, and hygiene care should be provided to the rectum and genital area at each change.

Checklist: Swallowing problems

- ☐ Many individuals with Alzheimer's disease lose the ability to swallow. Because this makes maintaining adequate nutrition difficult, it is often a sign that your loved one is in the last few months or weeks of life.

- ☐ Difficulties swallowing increase the risk of choking or of food going down the windpipe into the lungs, called aspiration. Aspiration pneumonia, which occurs when food or fluids are breathed into the lungs, can cause difficulty breathing. Aspiration pneumonia is a common cause of death for individuals with Alzheimer's disease.

- ☐ Help your loved one remember to swallow by gently stroking the person's neck in a downward motion and saying "swallow."

- ☐ Avoid the use of straws. Straws often make swallowing more difficult.

- ☐ Soft foods are best for individuals who have difficulty swallowing.

- ☐ Thin liquids and hot liquids are more difficult to swallow, so avoid them. Liquids can be thickened using Thick-It® or other thickening agents.

- ☐ If your loved one is unable to swallow but is otherwise still in good physical health, you may want to discuss artificial nutrition and hydration with the physician. Keep in mind, though, that tube feeding does not prevent aspiration, and it does not prolong life for people with Alzheimer's disease.

- ☐ If your loved one requires tube feeding due to an inability to swallow, they may not understand the purpose of feeding tubes or IV lines, so they may attempt to remove them, causing pain and risk of infection.

Checklist: Musculoskeletal problems

- ☐ At the end of life, individuals with Alzheimer's lose the ability to move independently. Therefore, the individual will not be able to walk or sit upright without assistance and will need help with all daily activities.

- ☐ Because the individual cannot move independently, they will primarily be bed-bound. To help prevent pressure ulcers, the individual should be rotated at least every 2 hours.

- ☐ If the person needs to move for some reason, you will need to learn how to lift the person safely. A care provider can give instructions for how to do this safely, help you move the person, or perform the lift for you. If you are helping move the person, do not lift the person by pulling on the person's arms or shoulders.

- ☐ If you give the person something to hold during the transfer or rotating process, such as a washcloth, they will be less likely to grab onto you or the furniture.

- ☐ Help the individual perform passive range-of-motion exercises for the arms and legs. A physician or other care provider can give you instructions for the best exercises and how often to perform them. These exercises can help prevent joint contractures, which occur when the muscles contract in such a way that it permanently shortens the muscle or joint. This causes joints to lock up and become immobile.

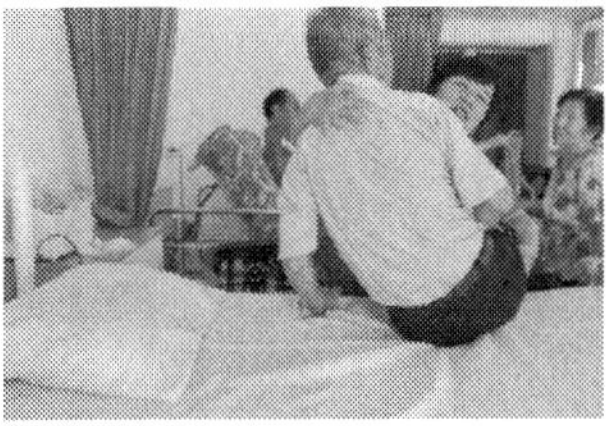

Credit: aodaodaodaod

- ☐ As the person loses musculoskeletal control, even the neck muscles will lose strength and will be unable to hold up the person's head. Make sure the person's head is always supported, especially during movement.

- ☐ Some individuals will develop myoclonus, in which the person's extremities or entire body jerks. This may look like a seizure, but the individual does not lose consciousness. Inform the physician immediately if this occurs.

Checklist: Urinary problems

- ☐ Incontinence, a lack of bladder control, may occur. There are several options for handling this.

- ☐ If the person is able to stand and walk with help, a regular toileting schedule may prevent episodes of incontinence.

- ☐ For individuals who are not mobile, a catheter tube placed in the bladder that allows urine to drain into a collection bag can help some people with incontinence problems.

- ☐ The area where the catheter enters the body must be kept clean daily to prevent infection, and the drainage bag must be emptied at least twice daily in addition to being kept properly positioned below the level of the person with the drainage tube unobstructed.

- ☐ When using a catheter, watch for any leaking around the catheter. Watch out for urine that contains blood or becomes cloudy or smelly. Watch for fever. Report any of these problems when you see them because they are signs of infection.

- ☐ If needed, incontinence pads can be used. Incontinence pads must be changed often, and the skin should be kept clean and dry to prevent skin breakdown.

- ☐ Water-repellent creams or sprays containing zinc oxide and silicone can help prevent or reduce skin irritation for people who wear incontinence pads.

- ☐ At the end of life, the kidneys may shut down. Coupled with dehydration, this often results in minimal urine production. If urine production is minimal, your loved one may require dialysis to remove toxins from the body.

Checklist: Increased susceptibility to infections

- ☐ Individuals with Alzheimer's disease are susceptible to a variety of infections.

- ☐ Pneumonia is a common infection because individuals with Alzheimer's disease have lost the ability to cough or cannot remember how to cough, so secretions and aspirated substances remain in the lungs and can become infected.

- ☐ Improper care of a urinary catheter for incontinence or long-term use of the catheter often results in urinary tract infections.

- If a foot or hand becomes wounded or cracks due to dry skin, the skin may develop an infection due to poor circulation and the inability to fight bacteria at the site.

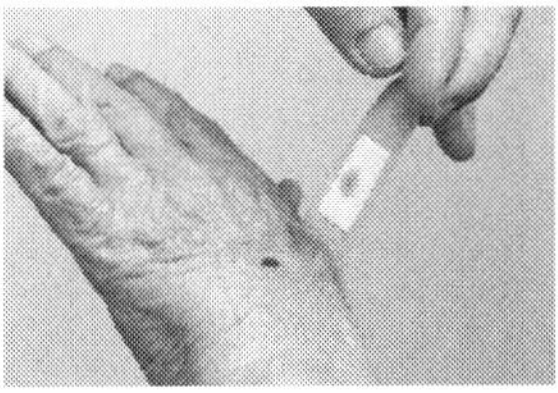

Credit: Toa55

- Signs of an infection in individuals with dementia often differ from other individuals. Signs and symptoms are more likely to be related to sudden behavioral changes than physical changes. Signs and symptoms may include:
    - Fever
    - Sudden increase in confusion
    - Falling
    - Decreased appetite
    - Pain
    - Paranoia or delusions
    - Delirium
    - Urinary incontinence
- If the person with Alzheimer's disease has trouble swallowing, typical oral medications to treat infections cannot be used. Antibiotics may need to be given via IV, but if the person does not understand why the tubes are in place, they may pull them out, creating another potential site of infection.
- Good oral hygiene can reduce the risk of respiratory infections.

- □ Avoid the use of a urinary catheter if possible, and use good hygiene practices in the genital area.
- □ Treat cuts and scrapes immediately by cleaning the cut and applying an antibiotic ointment.
- □ Consider having a medical professional administer influenza and pneumonia vaccines when appropriate.
- □ Aspiration pneumonia and infected pressure ulcers are two common causes of death in individuals with Alzheimer's disease.

Witnessing the physical and mental transformations wrought by end-of-life symptoms can be agonizing. Try anything you can to alleviate the suffering from these symptoms. You can find stories about personal experiences with an Alzheimer's disease patient dying online. This person's powerful story, which was originally published on the editorially independent news site Being Patient, is an example:

https://www.beingpatient.com/alzheimers-death/

In addition to finding and reading other people's stories, don't discount the need for professional counseling. Being witness to a loved one's death is a traumatic experience; dealing with the emotional effects of that is not something you should try to do alone.

Chapter 2: Palliative Care vs. Hospice Care

During the course of your loved one's disease, you may hear the terms "palliative care" and "hospice care" used by the medical team. Sometimes, it seems like they use these terms interchangeably, but they do not refer to the same type of care. What are the similarities and differences? In general, both palliative care and hospice care provide compassionate or comfort care for individuals with life-limiting illnesses. They both provide treatment to relieve pain and discomfort from symptoms, and they both provide aspects of care related to spiritual, emotional, and mental wellness.

However, palliative care and hospice care also have some very important differences. Palliative care should begin at the time of diagnosis and continue through the end of life. It does not depend on prognosis. In contrast, hospice care is reserved for individuals with a terminal illness who are not expected to live more than six months. Another difference is the option to continue curative treatments. With palliative care, treatments that are intended to cure the illness can continue. In contrast, with hospice care, curative treatments have failed and are not expected to improve the patient's life any longer. Therefore, all curative treatments related to the terminal illness are stopped during hospice care. More specific details about palliative care and hospice care are provided in the following sections.

Palliative Care

Palliative care does not focus on extending the life of the person but on improving and preserving that person's comfort and dignity. Palliative care seeks to maximize the person's quality of life both in its physical and mental health dimensions. It seeks to address end-of-life symptoms, such as pain, depression, fatigue, difficulty sleeping, and loss of appetite, as much as can be managed. The following checklist covers some basic facts about palliative care.

Checklist: Palliative care facts

- ☐ Palliative care is performed in a variety of settings:
  - Hospitals
  - Nursing homes
  - Outpatient care clinics
  - In the home
- ☐ Palliative care specialists treat people with a wide range of serious long-term illnesses. Patients need not be dying to receive palliative care, and any patient dealing with general discomfort and disability should receive palliative care.
- ☐ Palliative care specialists can help their patients and family understand their medical options.
- ☐ Palliative care provides support in four dimensions:
  - Physical comfort
  - Mental and emotional needs
  - Spiritual needs
  - Help with practical tasks
- ☐ Preserving physical comfort involves addressing many issues, including:
  - Pain
  - Breathing problems

   - Skin irritation
   - Digestive problems
   - Fatigue

- Providing for the person's mental and emotional needs involves addressing both generalized feelings of depression, anxiety, and distress and specific fears and concerns.

- Providing for the person's spiritual needs involves ensuring the person's religious requirements are met. It also may involve finding a sense of meaning and resolving personal conflicts that cause the person guilt and remorse.

- Practical help involves any task that needs to be done to provide relief to the person with Alzheimer's disease or to caregivers for that person. It could be doing chores around the house, running errands, or helping with activities of daily living.

- Medical personnel, family, and friends should provide palliative care in all interactions with the individual with Alzheimer's disease.

- Palliative care for patients with Alzheimer's disease involves creating a routine with physical and mental exercise and maintaining a calm, quiet, and properly lit environment. It also involves connecting with patients through the senses: touch, hearing, and smell, such as playing favorite music or providing them with pleasant and familiar smells.

- Insurance coverage for palliative care will depend on your benefits and treatment plan.

Hospice Care

The main goal of hospice care is to allow individuals to transition to the end of life with dignity, so the focus of hospice care is on comfort and support. Hospice care provides only comfort care, not treatment. Therefore, hospice care seeks not to cure illness but to manage pain and ease the effects of terminal illness on the person with the illness and on that person's family and other supporters, similar to palliative care. In the early stages of Alzheimer's disease, you should talk to your loved one about what they prefer in regard to end-of-life care, and this information should be spelled out in advance directive documents (See Long-Term Care Insurance, Power of Attorney, Wealth Management, and Other First Steps). This will likely be a very difficult conversation for both your loved one and your family, but it is important to know what your loved one would prefer. Many doctors and social workers do not recommend the use of feeding tubes, respirators, and other life-prolonging techniques in the advanced stages of Alzheimer's disease. However, this is a decision that your loved one will need to make for themselves through the use of a living will.

Hospice care will only begin when a doctor has agreed that the individual has six months or less left to live. This form of care will not provide aggressive medical treatment for the terminal illness but will instead provide pain and symptom management during the last months of life. However, treatment for non-terminal conditions can continue. For example, if your loved one with Alzheimer's disease also has diabetes, treatment for the diabetes will continue unchanged once your loved

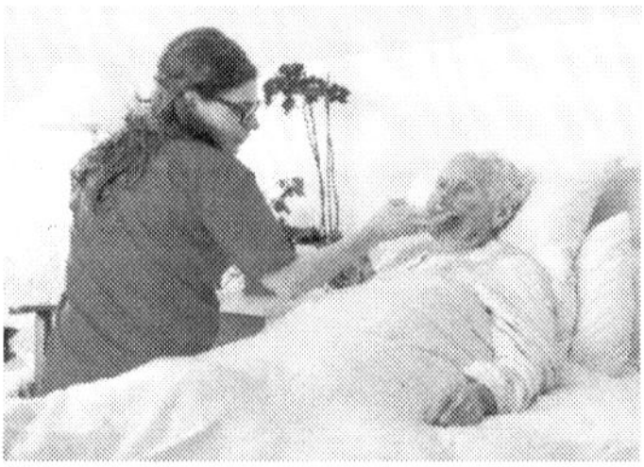

Credit: Lighthunter

one enters hospice care. Hospice can be done in your loved one's home or at a residential facility or hospital. Workers often include doctors, nurses, social workers, and spiritual counselors. Your hospice care provider will create a care plan that addresses each of your loved one's specific pain management and symptom control needs.

Hospice programs must meet requirements at both the state and federal levels. A hospice must meet state licensure requirements in order to deliver care. To maintain its license, it must continue to meet regulatory standards and pass periodic inspections. To receive approval for Medicare reimbursement, hospices must comply with relevant federal regulations and pass regular inspections to maintain this certification. The National Hospice and Palliative Care Organization works to ensure the quality of hospice care through a set of recommended standards called "Standards of Practice for Hospice Programs," and various voluntary accreditation organizations evaluate hospices according to standards such as the NHPCO's.

The following checklist outlines the basic hospice eligibility requirements. For eligible patients, costs for hospice care are typically covered by insurance, including Medicare and Medicaid.

Checklist: Hospice eligibility requirements

- ☐ The person must be entitled to Part A of Medicare.
- ☐ The person must be certified as being terminally ill by a physician (a primary care physician or hospice physician) with a prognosis of six or fewer months to live, assuming the disease runs its normal course. Patients of any age may receive hospice care.
- ☐ The patient and family must:
    - o Fully understand the prognosis.

- Agree to seek palliative care instead of seeking a cure.
- Provide informed consent.
- Choose the hospice benefit by completing and signing an election form.

☐ Medicare allows for a one-time visit by a physician, either the medical director of or employee of a hospice agency, to:

- Evaluate the individual's need for pain and symptom management.
- Counsel the individual regarding hospice and other care options.
- Advise the individual regarding advanced care planning.

☐ In order to be eligible to receive this service, a beneficiary must, in addition to meeting the terminal illness requirement, have not made a hospice election and not previously received pre-election hospice services.

The checklist below discusses some of the services hospice provides.

Checklist: Services provided by hospice

☐ Pain and symptom management and relief.

☐ Management of non-terminal conditions will continue unchanged.

☐ Counseling about the end-of-life process for both your loved one and family.

- ☐ Grief counseling for family members.
- ☐ A focus on the quality of life for the remaining time your loved one has.
- ☐ Increased focus on the emotional needs of your loved one.
- ☐ An emphasis on comfort in terms of pain relief, anxiety reduction, spiritual services, and overall care.

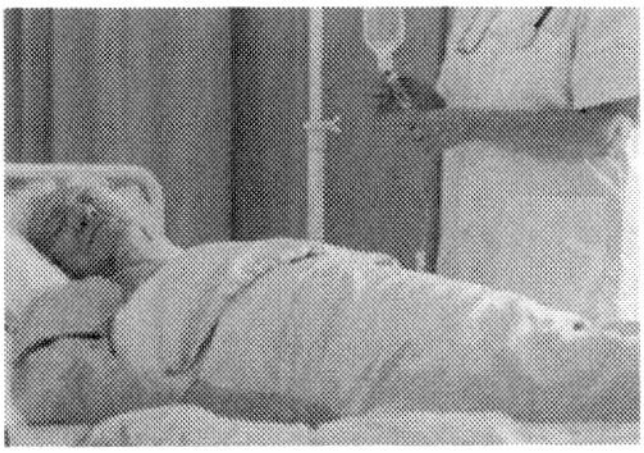

Credit: Photographee.eu

- ☐ Visits from doctors, nurses, counselors, dieticians, therapists, social workers, and spiritual counselors.
- ☐ A plan of care specific to your loved one's desires and needs.
- ☐ All medical supplies, equipment, and therapies provided as needed.
- ☐ Care in a home setting, as well as in long- or short-term care facilities and hospitals.
- ☐ Therapeutic massage.
- ☐ Music therapy and pet therapy.
- ☐ Relaxation technique training.
- ☐ Assistance with bathing and/or personal care.
- ☐ 24-hour-a-day on-call staff.
- ☐ Help to the family so that they may come to an acceptance of their loved one's condition.
- ☐ Access to support groups for family members.

- □ Help from social workers to facilitate access to resources within the community.
- □ Help from trained, compassionate volunteers who can provide support to your loved one and family members, as well as assist with daily tasks such as shopping or babysitting.
- □ Trained respite care for caregivers.

The checklist below covers the range of end-of-life care needs of people with Alzheimer's disease. Monitor whether these needs appear to be appropriately met for your loved one by hospice care or other caregivers by answering the questions in this checklist.

Checklist: End-of-life care needs and actions

- □ Is your loved one receiving enough stimulation? Remember to connect through the senses, such as touching your loved one's hand to reassure them that you are nearby. Speak to your loved one in a calm and natural voice. Play favorite music. Bringing pleasing scents close to your loved one such as a favorite flower or perfume.
- □ Is your loved one having difficulty breathing? Raise the head of the bed or raise the upper body with pillows.
- □ While eating and for 30 minutes after eating, is your loved one seated in a comfortable upright position to aid swallowing and digestion?
- □ Is self-feeding encouraged but assistance with eating provided as and when needed?

- ☐ Does your loved one ever appear to be dehydrated? Signs of dehydration include a number of symptoms—dry mouth, sleepiness and tiredness, thirst, headaches, constipation, and dizziness—that can be difficult to assess in someone with Alzheimer's disease, but check for dryness of skin and try to monitor how often your loved one urinates.

- ☐ Does it appear that your loved one is being encouraged to ingest an appropriate amount of fluids?

- ☐ Is your loved one being given an adequate toileting schedule? Are necessary incontinence products being used and are these incontinence products being changed regularly?

- ☐ Does your loved one appear to be losing too much weight? Weight loss for someone approaching the end of life is normal, but if you are concerned about your loved one's weight loss, seek the advice of a physician.

- ☐ Is your loved one being given regular changes in position to avoid circulation problems? Range of motion exercises are helpful for keeping your loved one's limbs and joints from becoming too rigid. To reposition your loved one yourself, use slow, gentle movements to relieve pressure areas, focusing on one part of the body at a time.

- ☐ Is your loved one being given proper cushioning to avoid pressure ulcers?

- ☐ Is your loved one's skin being kept clean and dry? If your loved one's skin appears clean but has some bruising, that might be a sign that washing isn't gentle enough. Rashes and bedsores are a sign that cleaning isn't frequent enough. If you wash your loved one, use as little force and friction as possible, washing the skin gently and blotting it dry as you go.

- ☐ Using lotion, gently massage your loved one's hands and feet.

- ☐ Are your loved one's teeth and mouth being kept clean? If your loved one is no longer eating or drinking, take care to keep the lips moist to continue to provide mouth care.

- ☐ Has your loved one suffered any cuts or scrapes, and have these been treated immediately?

- ☐ Is your loved one receiving vaccinations against the flu and pneumonia as often as necessary?

- ☐ Does your loved one show signs of pain and discomfort? These might include swelling, angry changes in skin color such as flushed skin, or facial expressions such grimacing or wincing. Ensure that proper pain control medications are used to relieve your loved one's discomfort.

- ☐ Does your loved show signs of distress such as anxiety or sleeping problems?

Chapter 3: Stopping End-of-Life Care

You may need to make the decision to stop end-of-life care for your loved one. If your loved one is unable to continue to live without artificial nutrition and hydration (ANH) or artificial respiration, then the decision to start, forego, or end such measures must be made. This is not euthanasia, the active ending of a life, but the cessation of efforts to sustain life through artificial measures. If your loved one with Alzheimer's disease is in the advanced stages of the disease, it will not be possible for your loved one to make this decision. Because the decision about whether to administer ANH or artificial respiration is an end-of-life decision, it is likely that Alzheimer's disease for your loved one will have progressed to the point that they are no longer mentally capable of making this or any other choice. This is why it's important to discuss this issue with your loved one early and record their wishes in advance directives.

When making decisions about advance directives, your loved one, your loved one's family, and your loved one's physician need to discuss the possible end-of-life scenarios and the specific choices each one involves. Make sure that your loved one fully understands these issues and makes clear, definite decisions regarding the choices involved in end-of-life care. Please involve mental health professionals you and your loved one trust, clergy from your loved one's faith community, and any other spiritual or mental health advisor who might be able to help your loved one make the necessary decisions. Once your loved one has recorded their wishes in their advance directives, make sure you refer to them when the time for end-of-life decisions arrives. In this way, you and your loved one's family will be aware of what your loved one wants before you face any hard choices, and you will be guided by that knowledge when you do have to make those choices.

Artificial Nutrition and Hydration (ANH)

Artificial nutrition and hydration become necessary when a patient is no longer capable of swallowing effectively enough to ingest the food and liquids necessary to sustain life. ANH may be administered on a short- or long-term basis, depending on the patient's specific circumstances. Replacement of liquids in a patient requiring ANH may be accomplished intravenously through an IV drip that transfers the necessary liquids directly into the bloodstream via a catheter tube inserted into a vein. Fluid replacement may also be accomplished through a process called hypodermoclysis, in which liquids are replaced subcutaneously, meaning beneath the skin. Feeding and hydration may be accomplished through a tube placed in the gastrointestinal tract; the entrance to this tube may be through either the nose or the stomach. When through the nose, this is called a nasogastric or NG tube. The NG tube goes through the nose and then down the throat and into the stomach; this tube is not usually used for more than four weeks and constitutes a short-term care option. The longer-term feeding solution is the gastric or G tube, also called a PEG tube, which goes directly into the stomach. For such a tube to work, the patient must be sedentary (not moving from the bed) long enough for the "feeding" and digestion to complete, and these feedings happen several times a day.

The use of a PEG tube is extremely restrictive, therefore, and the restrictive environment it creates for the patient lowers the patient's quality of life significantly. Additionally, short-term mortality rates for patients who go on PEG tubes are high. Also, studies reveal that the popular belief that use of such tubes prevents aspiration pneumonia (which results from substances from the mouth being breathed into the lungs) is mistaken; research has found that these tubes do not actually prevent aspiration pneumonia.

The checklist below discusses some of the issues involved in ANH.

Checklist: ANH issues and concerns

- ☐ High-quality palliative or hospice care aims to increase comfort and maintain a high quality of life for patients, but this is not the goal of ANH.

- ☐ ANH sustains life function at the expense of quality of life in terms of comfort and freedom of movement.

- ☐ ANH generally preserves life function at the lowest possible level.

- ☐ ANH must be administered only by qualified medical professionals in an appropriate healthcare environment.

- ☐ Studies do not show that ANH prevents aspiration pneumonia, so the risk of such pneumonia continues after the decision to administer ANH.

- ☐ Short-term mortality rates following the administration of ANH, meaning death of patients soon after being given ANH, are significantly high.

- ☐ Catheters may cause infection at the point of insertion.

- ☐ The insertion of an NG tube may cause choking and considerable discomfort after placement.

- ☐ An NG tube may become misplaced; cause pneumonia through fluid entering the lungs; and cause damage to the nasal and esophageal (throat) passages and to the stomach, which may lead to acute or chronic bleeding.

- □ A G tube requires the patient to be anesthetized during placement, and so the risks of anesthesia are a concern.
- □ A G tube may cause nausea, infection, gastrointestinal bleeding, diarrhea, or aspiration pneumonia. It can block or perforate the bowel.
- □ Because a confused patient may attempt to pull out an NG tube or a G tube, the patient may need to be restrained if either tube is administered.
- □ Hand feeding, also called assisted oral feeding, is an alternative to tube feeding that is potentially less risky for a patient with Alzheimer's disease or other dementia.

Artificial Respiration

Artificial respiration involves the use of a ventilator. This is a tube that is inserted either down the throat or directly into the throat via a tracheotomy, which is known as intubation. Artificial respiration may be required in the short term when an illness such as pneumonia requires a patient to need assistance with breathing while combating the disease. But long-term artificial respiration may be required to sustain the life function of patients who, through chronic (prolonged) illness or weakness, are no longer capable of breathing on their own.

As with ANH, artificial respiration is invasive, restricts movement, and carries risks of its own, and so the use of artificial respiration involves a significant decrease in the quality of life of the patient.

The checklist below discusses some of the issues involved with artificial respiration.

Checklist: Artificial respiration issues and concerns

- ☐ A ventilator will not stop the dying process; it only provides a way for patients to breathe and does not treat or cure the illness or other problem that led to the ventilator being administered.
- ☐ The administration of a ventilator may require additional testing such as a blood test and X-rays to administer safely.
- ☐ Administration of a ventilator carries the risk of infection.
- ☐ The ventilator does not cause patients pain, but some patients may not like the feeling of the tube in their throat.
- ☐ The ventilator prevents the patient from talking because of its position with respect to the vocal cords.
- ☐ Patients may need to be sedated to decrease discomfort or so that they do not try to breathe on their own (thus interfering with the functioning of the ventilator).
- ☐ It is difficult to know when it is administered how long a ventilator may be required.
- ☐ Physicians will endeavor to keep the patient's time on the ventilator brief, slowly reducing the patient's dependence on the ventilator in a process known as "weaning," but this is not always possible to do.
- ☐ The decision to remove a ventilator is stressful and emotional for many people, so once administered, the decision to remove a ventilator may be especially difficult.

Ethical and Emotional Issues

The dilemma that ANH and ventilators present is a fundamental conflict between sustaining the individual's life function and sustaining that person's quality of life. ANH and artificial respiration represent extraordinary measures to preserve the basic biological functions of a person at the cost of the things that may make life worth living in that person's eyes. The ability to move freely, to speak, to remain conscious—all of these may be extremely restricted or even impossible given the specific measures involved and the patient's particular circumstances. Additionally, as outlined above, there are physical risks involved with such measures. Infections and other complications may result that create new problems to be addressed, potentially through even more treatments and invasive measures.

Given these concerns, the decision to resort to ANH or artificial respiration must be considered carefully. If your loved one has a Do Not Resuscitate (DNR) order, this forbids medical and emergency personnel from performing CPR in the event that your loved one's breathing stops. However, a DNR does not forbid the use of a ventilator. Even if your loved one has a DNR in place, you must discuss the issue of ventilators with your loved one. As early as possible, discuss these end-of-life choices with your loved one and understand as much as possible what your loved one wishes in this regard. This understanding should be communicated in the presence of and understood equally by you, your loved one, your loved one's family, and your loved one's physician so that all involved have a shared view of your loved one's final wishes. Advance directives can prevent misunderstanding or confusions by preserving your loved one's decisions in written, legal form.

Remember that the law does not prevent the ending of medical measures that do not cure or control an illness. ANH and artificial respiration measures do not cure or control illness. They only allow hydration, nutrition, or respiration to continue. The decision to forego or end such measures is not illegal if it is made by the patient or someone empowered to make health decisions on behalf of the patient in the event that the patient is no longer capable of making such decisions. It is a moral, ethical, and emotional issue, but not necessarily a legal one. Healthcare staff must respect the loved one's wishes if expressed in an advance directive or through a healthcare proxy empowered to act on the loved one's behalf. However, in the absence of such directives, disagreements regarding the administration of ANH or artificial respiration may require a second opinion from another healthcare provider, speaking to the ethics committee of the healthcare facility, or arbitration to resolve.

The checklist below discusses some of the questions to answer regarding the decision to forego or end ANH or artificial respiration measures.

Checklist: Questions concerning ANH and artificial respiration

- ☐ What are my loved one's expressed wishes regarding ANH or artificial respiration?
- ☐ What may my loved one's quality of life be without ANH or artificial respiration measures to prolong my loved one's life?
- ☐ If a breathing or feeding tube is recommended by a physician treating my loved one, what is the reason? How long will the tube need to be used? Is use of the tube likely to be permanent?
- ☐ Will my loved one need to be restrained or sedated to allow proper functioning of the tube?

- ☐ Will my loved one need to be administered antibiotics to prevent infection while on the tube?
- ☐ Does the medical and healthcare staff treating my loved one know my loved one's decisions regarding ANH or artificial respiration?
- ☐ Does the staff agree with my loved one's expressed wishes regarding ANH or artificial respiration? (Again, their agreement is not necessarily required, but in the absence of advance directives or other such indications of your loved one's clear wishes, disagreements with staff about ANH or artificial respiration may require the involvement of additional parties to resolve.)
- ☐ If my loved one has no advance directives and has not clearly expressed their wishes regarding ANH or artificial respiration to a healthcare proxy, and there is disagreement regarding the decision to avoid or end such treatment, how will this issue be resolved?

The decision to stop artificial nutrition, hydration, or respiration—or to forego such measures entirely—is highly emotional. It's one of the most difficult decisions you or your loved one may need to make. If it falls to you, remember your loved one's choices in this regard as you understand them, and also remember what your loved one's personal values are. Studies suggest that the process of dying from a lack of nutrition or from dehydration is not painful for elderly

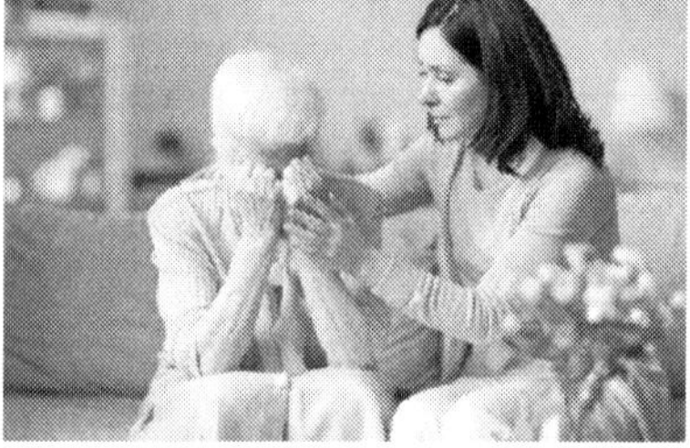

Credit: Pressmaster

patients. Remember that to get to the point where artificial measures of prolonging life function become necessary, the patient's bodily function has already deteriorated past the point of the patient's own ability to sustain it. Artificial measures will not make your loved one feel better or stronger, and they will not reverse the process of deterioration. What would your loved one want? What does your loved one value more: life at any cost or quality of life? Keep your loved one's wishes and values in view, and you'll make the best decision you can under the circumstances.

Chapter 4: Grieving

Grieving is a necessary process for accepting a painful loss. Grieving for a loved one with Alzheimer's disease is especially complicated because the disease lasts for many years and because, due to the nature of the disease and the mental decline it causes, you begin losing your loved one long before death. It's important to be aware of the signs and stages of grieving because they are a part of the process of caring for a loved one with Alzheimer's disease.

The Stages of Grief

The psychologist Elisabeth Kübler-Ross in 1969 posed the idea that the grieving process can generally be divided into five stages. You have probably encountered this idea already. It is a very commonly used model for understanding grief. According to Kübler-Ross, the five stages of grief are denial, anger, bargaining, depression, and acceptance.

No one deals with loss and grief the same way, however, so although the Kübler-Ross model is helpful for a general understanding of the emotions and reactions that attend grief for most people, remember that everyone is different, and that includes you. Don't try to fit your emotions and reactions into a preexisting model or framework. Try instead to be aware of your emotions and reactions. If you notice that you are acting in accordance with a model like the Kübler-Ross stages—you are acting in denial, for example, or bargaining or getting angry to

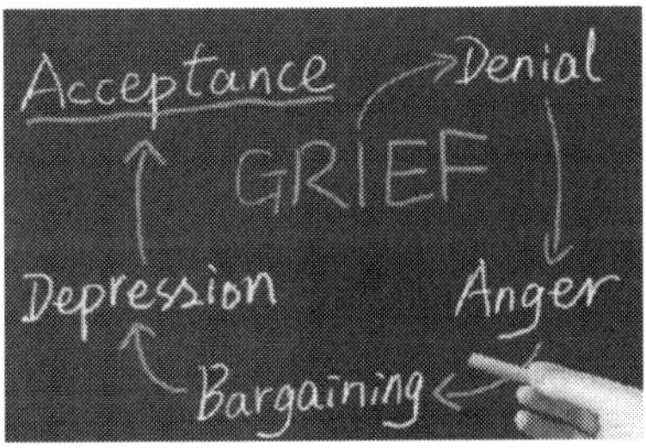

Credit: Raywoo

avoid dealing directly with your loss—you may understand your own emotions better and why you are reacting the way you do. The Kübler-Ross stages can also help you understand the behavior of others in response to grief and know why they are acting the way they do. Be patient and compassionate, both with yourself and with others. Sometimes even inappropriate behavior is part of the process, and no one grieves on the same timetable and in the same way. Recognize that, and let empathy (understanding what others feel) as well as sympathy (sharing in what others feel) be your guide.

The checklist below describes each stage of grief according to Kübler-Ross.

Checklist: Kübler-Ross stages of grief

- ☐ Denial, in which the grieving person tries to push away the reality of the loss
- ☐ Anger, in which the grieving person lashes out in an attempt to overcome the reality of the loss through finding a target to blame
- ☐ Bargaining, in which the grieving person tries to find ways to deal with loss as a negotiation that can be controlled
- ☐ Depression, in which the grieving person gives way to the overwhelming sadness of the loss
- ☐ Acceptance, in which the grieving person becomes able to accept the reality of the loss and move past it

Grieving for a Loved One with Alzheimer's Disease

Your loved one with Alzheimer's disease will progress through various stages of decline over the course of the disease, and every person with Alzheimer's disease experiences these stages differently. Two people with Alzheimer's disease may move through stages of the illness in a different order and may move back and forth between different stages in different ways. Although there is a general progression to the cognitive and physical decline that Alzheimer's disease causes, your loved one's experience with Alzheimer's disease will in various ways be unique.

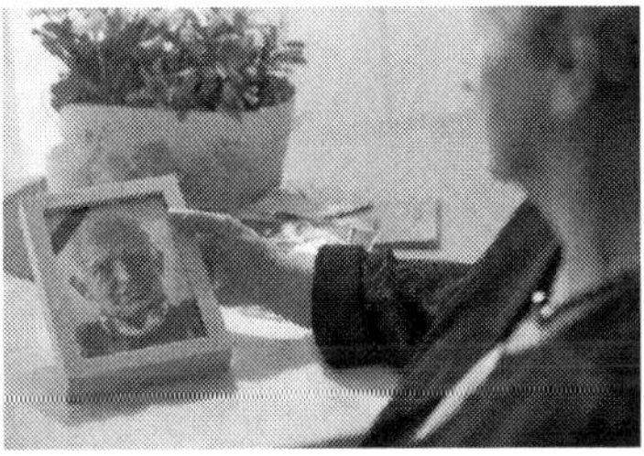

Credit: Photographee.eu

The same is true with grief. You may experience grief in ways that are right for you but might not seem right to others because you may not seem to show the symptoms of grief, such as sadness or anger or guilt, in ways that other people recognize. You may return to particular stages of grief, such as depression, many times, or stay in a particular stage for longer than seems normal to others. You may experience multiple stages at once—anger and denial, for example. No one goes through the grieving process the same way. This is true of all grief.

What makes grieving for a loved one with Alzheimer's disease particularly complicated is that you may begin grieving for your loved one well before your loved one actually dies. Grief involves loss. Death is one type of traumatic loss that causes people to grieve. But losing a loved one to Alzheimer's disease is also a loss that is like death in that what you lose about your loved one—the recognition in their eyes, the memories you share, the history you've built up between each other—can't be recovered except perhaps in brief flashes. This loss is in many ways as irrevocable and heartbreaking as death. What many people go through in caring for a loved one with Alzheimer's disease is called anticipatory grief, which is the realization that in ways both large and small you are gradually losing your loved one.

Alzheimer's disease progresses over a long course of time, and this is another way that grieving for a loved one with Alzheimer's disease is complicated. Over the course of your loved one's mental and physical decline, you may find yourself grieving in many ways and at many different times. Because grief can have severe emotional effects as well as physical effects—including but not limited to fatigue, insomnia, weight fluctuations, nausea, and aches and pains—recognizing when and how you are grieving is a part of the self-care you must maintain as you care for your loved one and deal with the loss of your loved one over time. Understand as well that you may long for your loved one's death at times, and you may be relieved when it finally happens. This is normal. You should not feel guilty for feeling this way. However, recognize that guilt is often a significant part of grief. If you understand that guilt over breaking down or just wanting it all to be over is a common part of grieving for many people, it may help you come to terms with your feelings faster.

The checklist below covers some facts about grieving that are helpful to remember.

Checklist: Facts about grieving

- ☐ You can't ignore your grief. Like all powerful emotions that are repressed, feelings of deep grief will have a strong effect on you even if you try to push them down or away. It's best to admit your grief, even if it's painful.

- ☐ You might need to be strong for your loved one or for others around you, but you can't always be. If you're overwhelmed at times, that's normal and healthy.

- ☐ You have to be able to feel what you feel. Your grief may not look right to others. But you need to experience and show grief in your own way.

- ☐ There is no set time limit on grief. Some people have an expectation that there is a particular period of time—a year, maybe, or even just a few months or a few weeks—during which grief is acceptable, but then people should just get over it. But different people grieve for different lengths of time.

- ☐ You may not go through the grieving process just once and that's it. You may find yourself going through the process of grieving several times.

- ☐ Your grieving process might not feel like a process at all, and that's okay. It may feel chaotic or formless. Don't expect that grief is going to be like checking off items in a list because it may not work that way or feel that way at all.

- ☐ Grieving and depression can be very much alike, but while grieving is a natural process, prolonged depression is a serious health issue that may need to be treated if you find it to be unmanageable.

The following checklist covers some ways to work through grief honestly and preserve your health as much as possible.

Checklist: Working through grief

- ☐ Face how you feel. Be honest and open with yourself. Look for creative ways to express your feelings.
- ☐ Don't let anyone else tell you what you feel.
- ☐ Talk to other people, in particular family members or friends who are your best source of support.
- ☐ Don't isolate yourself. Look for sources of support and comfort.
- ☐ Take care of yourself, including taking care of your physical as well as emotional needs.
- ☐ Take care of others, including friends and family. Helping others can give you meaning and focus when you need it the most.
- ☐ Pay attention to the grieving process of others and look for ways to help one another through the pain.
- ☐ Remember the good times with your loved one and cherish those memories.
- ☐ Talk to psychologists, therapists, grief counselors, and other support professionals.
- ☐ Watch yourself for signs of depression, such as prolonged and unmanageable feelings of hopelessness, guilt, and self-loathing.
- ☐ Seek professional help immediately if depression drives you to thoughts of suicide or self-harm, you sincerely wish that you had died instead, or you experience an inability to resume the normal activities of daily life after a number of weeks have passed.

Preparing for the Death of a Parent

If your loved one with Alzheimer's disease is a parent, grief can be especially complicated. It may not be possible to do some of the things children often do to say goodbye to their parents, such as finally saying long-unspoken things out loud or simply reminiscing about good times, because your parent will likely not understand you. Dementia typically takes away much of what made the parent a parent well before physical death occurs. However, preparing for the death of a parent with Alzheimer's disease is still a necessary part of making your peace with the event. The following checklist can help you do this.

Checklist: Preparing for the death of a parent with Alzheimer's disease

- ☐ Say what you need to say. Maybe your parent can understand you, maybe not. But say it anyway. Don't hold back from saying all the things to your parent that you have always wanted to say.
- ☐ Do reminisce as well. Tell stories involving you and your parent. You can still form a connection with your dying parent in spite of the dementia. Remember that you connect through the senses. By hearing your voice, seeing your face, and holding your hand, your parent can still connect with you.
- ☐ Remember to take care of yourself. Don't neglect your own needs physically, emotionally, or mentally. Take time out for your own life and care for your own health.
- ☐ If you have prepared legal documents with your parent in advance of the end of life (which with a parent with dementia is especially necessary to do

as early as possible following the diagnosis), be sure to have the most recent copy of all legal documents relevant to your parent's situation gathered together in a secure and easily accessed place. These include:

- o Trusts
- o Wills
- o Advance directives
- o Durable powers of attorney, both medical and financial

□ Honor your parent by carrying out their wishes. This includes attempting to avoid strife with family members and others over estate and other end-of-life issues. It may not be possible to avoid such conflicts, but try not to start or add to them with your own actions.

□ Be watchful for anticipatory grief and seek help if necessary. Signs of anticipatory grief include imagining your parent's death, thinking about the aftermath, and increasing concern for the parent. These are all normal responses to a parent approaching the end of life, but if you find yourself overwhelmed by the feelings these anticipatory responses evoke, turn to sources of support.

Also from Omega Press

Manage Your Stress and Your Fears

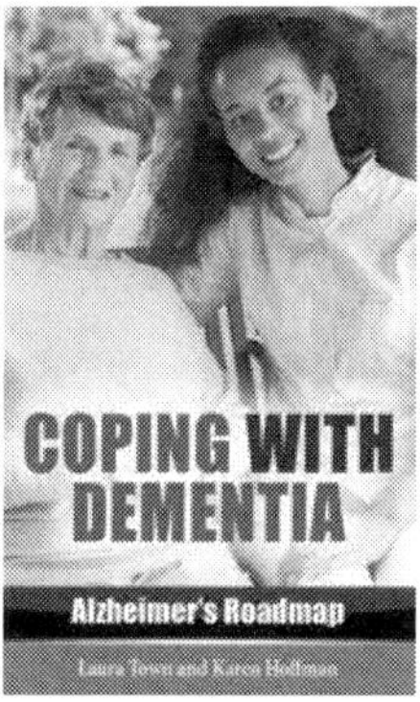

Coping with Dementia provides answers to the following questions and more:

- **How can I help my loved one following their diagnosis?** Learn how to help your loved one work through their day-to-day functional challenges as well as the complex emotions they have about their diagnosis.
- **What do we tell family and friends?** Consider how others in your loved one's life will react to their diagnosis and find ways to engage them in the caregiving process.
- **How will providing care to my loved one affect me?** Read about positive and negative aspects of caregiving, and learn strategies to care for yourself as well as your loved one.
- **How do I ensure my loved one is receiving proper care?** Learn how to pick a facility and monitor the care your loved one receives when their needs outgrow your capabilities.
- **Is there audio for this book?** Yes, you can find it here: https://www.audible.com/pd/Coping-with-Dementia-Alzheimers-Roadmap-Audiobook/B0815C8J74

Chapter 5: Burial or Cremation

When your loved one dies, in addition to handling all the emotions that come with that event, you will have to consider the arrangements necessary to either bury or cremate your loved one's remains. Of course, such arrangements themselves carry a strong emotional weight of their own. It can seem hateful and even unfair that you have to contend with such matters, but it must be done.

Getting a Death Certificate

You will need to register your loved one's death to obtain a death certificate. This checklist gives you the basic steps.

Checklist: Obtaining a death certificate

- ☐ Preparing and filing the death certificate is done by the funeral home, cremation organization, or other person in charge of the deceased person's remains.
- ☐ Preparing the certificate requires gathering personal information from family members, which varies by state but typically involves details such as full name, address, birth date, birthplace, the name and birthplace of the decedent's parents, Social Security number, and the date, place, and time of death.
- ☐ The death certificate requires the signature of a doctor, medical examiner, or coroner.
- ☐ The process of obtaining the death certificate must be completed within three to ten days, depending on state law.

- ☐ For death certificate ordering information, visit your state government's website.
- ☐ A fee is associated with obtaining copies of the death certificate.

Autopsy

An autopsy is still considered the gold standard for a definitive diagnosis of Alzheimer's disease. Although physicians can diagnose Alzheimer's disease before death with 90% accuracy, a brain autopsy is still the only definitive diagnosis available. Therefore, some families choose to have a brain autopsy performed on their loved one after death. The brain autopsy can provide helpful information for family members who want an accurate family medical history. Most medical examiners or coroners will only provide a brain autopsy upon request rather than a full autopsy for patients with Alzheimer's disease.

Usually, you will need to discuss your desires with your loved one's physician before your loved one's death to make arrangements for a brain autopsy after death. Most states do not require an autopsy for individuals with a known terminal illness, so it will be up to you to request an autopsy and make arrangements for it with your loved one's physician. In some states, physicians may not provide or arrange autopsies upon request. Instead, you may need to hire a private coroner for the autopsy at your own expense. Fees for an autopsy can range from free to $2,000 or more. An autopsy may be performed free of charge if your loved one died in a hospital or if your loved one was part of a research study on Alzheimer's disease. A private autopsy will be much more expensive, and autopsies are generally not covered by insurance. Therefore, you will need to decide if an autopsy and definitive diagnosis are worth the expense.

Another way to arrange for an autopsy and brain donation for research is through joining one of the national

Alzheimer's Disease Research Center studies. You will need to register your loved one for the study well before death, and the research center will follow your loved one's clinical progress throughout his or her life. Upon death, the research center will provide a brain only autopsy and will preserve your loved one's brain to help further research on Alzheimer's disease and other dementias. Without being part of one of these studies, it is very difficult to find any group who will accept a brain donation for research.

Planning for What Your Loved One Wants

Although many people do not pre-plan funeral arrangements, strongly consider making such "pre-need" arrangements with your loved one while it is still possible for your loved one to make decisions in this regard. When your loved one has expressed their wishes regarding funeral arrangements, you may approach a funeral home to begin the planning process. Search online for a funeral home directory to find one near you, or consider starting at www.funerals.org, the website of the Funeral Consumers Alliance. You might also consult the Federal Trade Commission's guide to shopping for funeral services. Whatever way you choose to start the process, if you plan the funeral now, you won't be burdened by having to make such arrangements immediately after your loved one has died. Your loved one may also consider a pre-paid burial plan. Pre-paid arrangements for burial or cremation dispose of the cost of such arrangements while your loved one is still alive and help ensure that this cost does not fall on anyone else after your loved one's death.

The checklist below covers some immediate questions to consider. These questions may or may not be appropriate for your loved one depending on cultural preferences. There are many different cultures in this country and around the world, and each culture may have its own preferences and customs regarding death, burial, cremation, and funeral services. Understanding and applying every cultural consideration is beyond the scope of this book, but hopefully these questions can get you started in the right direction.

Checklist: Immediate questions about burial and cremation

- □ Does your loved one want cremation or burial?
- □ Does your loved one want a direct burial, in which the fancy casket, viewing/visitation/wake, funeral service, and formal procession to the burial site are omitted?
- □ Does your loved one want a traditional, full-service burial that includes a casket suitable for viewing, some sort of viewing/visitation/wake, a funeral service, and a formal procession to the burial site?
- □ How elaborate does your loved one want the funeral to be?
- □ What religious services, if any, does your loved one require?
- □ Does your loved one have any particular wishes for the funeral?
- □ Does your loved one want to be buried or have their ashes scattered in a particular place?
- □ How does your loved one intend to pay for whatever end-of-life arrangement they desire?
- □ Will your loved one consider pre-paying for their chosen arrangement?

Direct Burial or Cremation

If your loved one chooses direct (immediate) cremation, then after death your loved one's body will be cremated without being embalmed. The cremated remains will be placed in an urn or similar container and given to the family or buried in a funeral plot if that is the desire your loved one has expressed.

If your loved one chooses direct (immediate) burial, then there usually won't be a viewing or visitation. Because your loved one will not be viewed, there is no need for embalming the body. There may be a funeral service at the burial site, but there does not need to be if that is not what your loved one wants. If your family would like a viewing before the cremation, some funeral homes will allow you to rent a casket for the viewing.

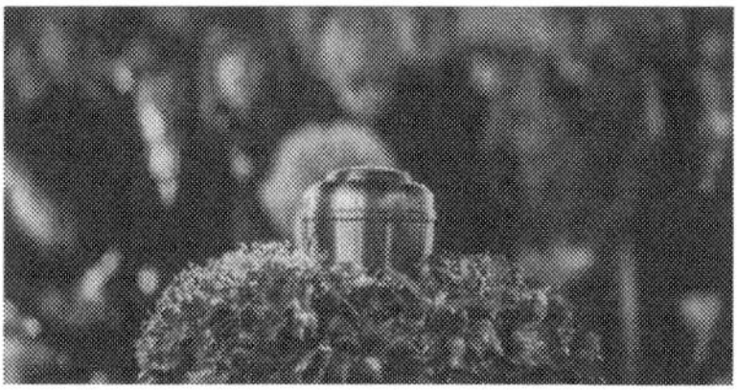

Credit: Anze Furlan

Another option other than burial or cremation is donation of the body for medical purposes. A school could use the body for study and research. A hospital may use parts of the body for study and research or for transplants and other life-saving medical procedures. Research into Alzheimer's disease is the best hope for one day finding a cure, and a medical donation may assist in such research. These arrangements must be made before death, and it is often very difficult to find an institution to take the body, so if your loved one wants their body donated, these arrangements should be made as soon as possible.

The checklist below covers the primary concerns involved in immediate burial or cremation.

Checklist: Concerns of direct burials or cremations

- ☐ For either direct burial or cremation, the funeral home will charge a basic services fee.
- ☐ Both direct burial and cremation involve a fee for transportation and care of the body.
- ☐ For cremation, there may be a fee, whether the funeral home has an on-site crematory or uses an off-site crematory service.
- ☐ The funeral home will provide a container for the body to be cremated in.
- ☐ The family will need to purchase or provide an urn or other container for the cremated remains.
- ☐ For direct burial, a casket or other suitable container must be purchased for the body.
- ☐ For burial of the body or cremated remains, there must be provision for a burial site, including reserving the lot or crypt, opening the lot or crypt, providing a grave liner if necessary (which prevents cave-ins and is typical for burial services), providing a marker or monument, and providing for ongoing grave maintenance.
- ☐ If there is to be a service at the burial site, there is typically a fee involved.

Traditional Burial

If your loved one chooses a traditional, full-service burial, then the body will be embalmed or other such arrangements will be made to make the body suitable for viewing or visitation. Of course, the funeral may also be closed casket, but typically in a traditional burial there will be a visitation, viewing, or wake of some kind, usually the day before or the day of burial. There also likely will be a funeral service, or some families might call this a memorial service or celebration of life service. A traditional burial involves more elaborate arrangements than either immediate burial or cremation and so tends to be more expensive.

The checklist below covers primary concerns involved in a burial or cremation involving a traditional funeral.

Checklist: Concerns of traditional funerals

- ☐ For a traditional funeral, the funeral home will charge a basic services fee.

- ☐ A traditional funeral involves a fee for transportation and care of the body.

- ☐ Typically, the body will be embalmed and dressed for viewing. The family will need to provide an outfit for the individual.

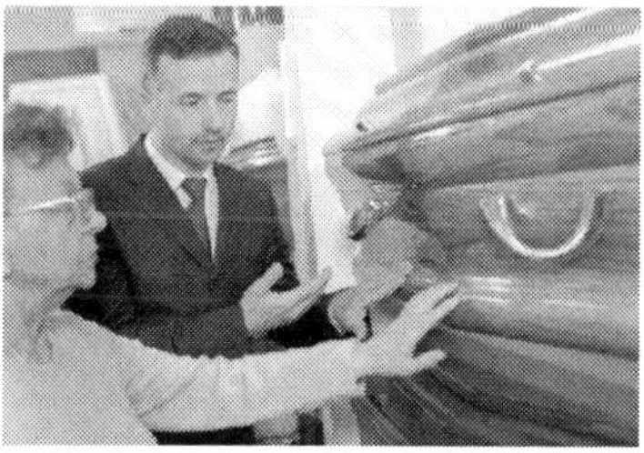

Credit: Phovoir

- ☐ A casket or other suitable container must be purchased for the body, unless the body is to be cremated following the funeral service, in which case the family will need to purchase or provide an urn or other suitable container for the cremated remains.

- ☐ A rental fee must be paid for the viewing or visitation at the funeral home. If the viewing or visitation is to be elsewhere such as in a person's home, there may be a cost involved in transporting the body to and from that location.

- ☐ It must be decided whether the viewing is to be public or private.
- ☐ A fee might be involved in the funeral service, whether it is held at the funeral home or in a place of worship. For a place of worship, although there may be no fee to a member of that congregation, typically a donation is still expected.
- ☐ It must be decided when the funeral or memorial service is to be performed and whether the body is to be present.
- ☐ The hearse or other vehicle used to transport the body to the burial site, as well as any vehicles the funeral home provides for the use of the family of the deceased, will have to be paid for.
- ☐ A fee is typically involved in providing the graveside service at the burial site.
- ☐ As with a direct burial or the burial of cremated remains, there must be provision for a burial site, including the lot or crypt, opening the lot or crypt, providing a grave liner if necessary (which prevents cave-ins and is typical for burial services), providing a marker or monument, and providing for ongoing grave maintenance.
- ☐ A funeral involving cremated remains can include any or all of the elements of a traditional funeral: visitation, wake, and church services. These can be prior to cremation or with the cremated remains present. The cremated remains may be buried in a cemetery.

Checklist: Planning a funeral

- ☐ If your loved one desired a traditional visitation, funeral, and graveside service, the family is typically involved in planning these services.
- ☐ The family, funeral home, and officiant will need to choose a date for the visitation and funeral. This will depend on when the funeral home can have the body ready and the availability of the desired facility, such as a church or funeral home.
- ☐ The visitation can be the night before the funeral, the same day before the funeral, or both. It can be at the funeral home, the church or other facility, or in a home.
- ☐ The visitation often involves a receiving line where individuals can share their condolences with immediate family.
- ☐ There may be a time of sharing during the visitation, funeral, or luncheon after the funeral.
- ☐ Pictures and other memorabilia are often on display for the visitation and funeral, and the family will need to prepare these displays if desired. A slideshow of pictures of the person's life may also be created and played at the visitation or funeral. Preparation of these items can start long before the individual dies.
- ☐ A bulletin that includes a picture of the individual, the obituary, and other information will need to be designed and printed. The funeral home often helps with this process.

- ☐ If desired, an obituary or death notice may be printed in the local paper or posted online by the funeral home.

- ☐ An order of service for the funeral needs to be prepared. This often depends on the individual's religious beliefs and traditions and may involve readings, music, and a message. Individuals involved with the service will need to be notified.

- ☐ If a graveside service is desired, the order of service for that will also need to be prepared in conjunction with the funeral home and officiant.

- ☐ A luncheon or other meal may be provided after the funeral or graveside service. Although this responsibility may fall on the family, it is often provided by friends of the deceased individual.

Chapter 6: Handling Your Loved One's Estate

When your loved one dies, your loved one's property is distributed according to the terms set out in your loved one's will. If your loved one had no will, then your loved one's property is distributed according to the terms of probate law for your loved one's state of residence. Estate planning, including the establishment of a durable power of attorney, a last will and testament, and a trust, is covered extensively in the book *Advance Directives, Durable Power of Attorney, Wills, and Other Legal Considerations*. We won't recap the full contents of that book here, but we will briefly touch on what you will need to consider immediately following the death of your loved one. Estate and other legal planning should be performed as early as possible with your loved one to ensure that their wishes are properly understood and respected. Additionally, because the laws and procedures governing estate distribution, disbursement of death benefits, and payment of debts vary by state, know what your loved one's state of residence requires.

The checklist below covers the basic things you need to do after your loved one dies, but be sure to consult the appropriate legal advice as necessary.

Checklist: Concerns regarding a loved one's estate, debts, and death benefits after death

- ☐ If your loved one has an estate plan, that should answer the questions of who has been appointed as administrator or executor of the estate and how your loved one's assets should be distributed.

- ☐ If your loved one had no estate plan, no will, and no indication of who should administrate the estate, probate court will appoint an estate administrator, who will be called the executor for the remainder of this checklist.
- ☐ The executor will collect all of the loved one's assets, pay creditors and debts, and distribute the remaining assets after the payment of debts to the loved one's beneficiaries as named in the will, or according to state law in the case of the absence of a will.
- ☐ The collection of assets will involve an inventory of all the assets of the loved one, including all their property and belongings.
- ☐ In the event that your loved one has no estate plan and the estate is small, probate court might not be necessary. Know the law regarding estate size for your loved one's state of residence.
- ☐ Unresolved debts incurred by your loved one will be paid out of their assets.
- ☐ After your loved one's debts are paid, the remainder of their assets go to their beneficiaries as named in the will or according to state law.
- ☐ An estate tax will be levied on any assets distributed to beneficiaries. There may be other taxes necessary, such as probate tax and various state and federal taxes, including income tax.
- ☐ For payment of death benefits, a death certificate will need to be obtained.

- ☐ The laws for obtaining a death certificate vary by state. Know the law for obtaining a death certificate in your loved one's state of residence.
- ☐ Obtain multiple copies of the death certificate.
- ☐ In addition to life insurance, there might be other benefits for which your loved one's survivors are eligible, such as Social Security.

Conclusion

The final stage of caring for a loved one with Alzheimer's disease is often emotionally painful for the family. Providing physical, emotional, and spiritual support for the individual requires gentleness, patience, and significant time. However, this can also be a time to make a few final meaningful memories with your loved one, knowing that you did all you could to make their last days the best they could be. Even though those last days are hard, you will never regret the time and care you gave to your loved one.

About the Authors

Laura Town

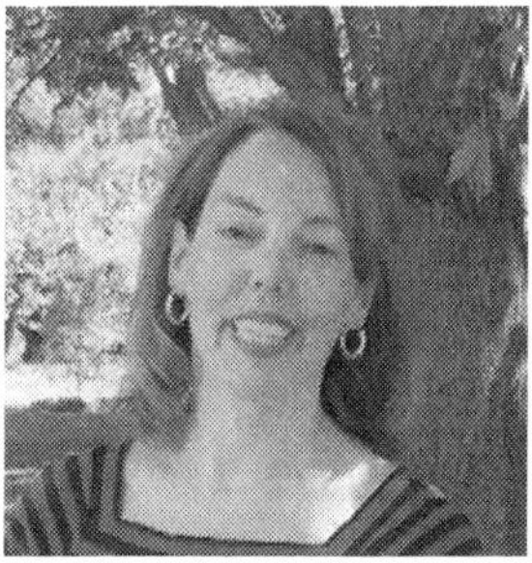

Laura Town has authored numerous publications of special interest to the aging population. She has expertise in the field of finance as a co-author on Finance: Foundations of Financial Institutions and Management published by John Wiley and Sons, and she has contributed to several online nursing courses and texts. She has also written for the American Medical Writers Association, and her work has been published by the American Society of Journalists and Authors. As an editor, Laura has worked with Pearson Education, Prentice Hall, McGraw-Hill Higher Education, John Wiley and Sons, and the University of Pennsylvania to create both on-ground and online courses and texts. She is the past president of the Indiana chapter of the American Medical Writers Association.

Karen Hoffman

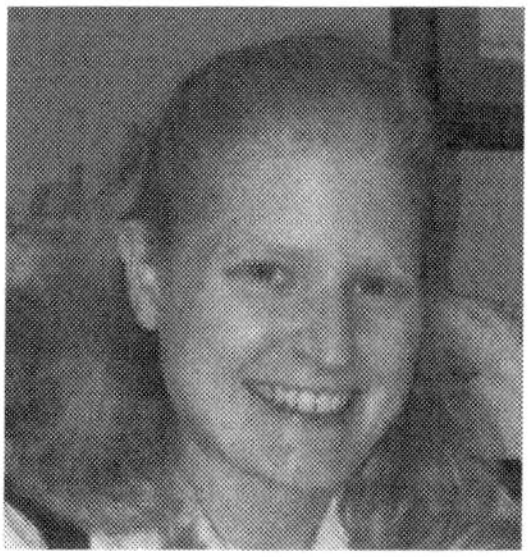

Karen Hoffman received her Ph.D. in Pharmacology from the Department of Pharmacology and Experimental Neurosciences at the University of Nebraska Medical Center in Omaha, NE, where she was the recipient of an American Heart Association fellowship and several regional and national awards for her research on G protein-coupled receptor signaling in airways. She then pursued post-doctoral research projects at the University of North

Carolina-Chapel Hill and the University of Kansas Medical Center, again receiving fellowships from the PhRMA Foundation and the American Heart Association, respectively. She has published research in the American Journal of Pathology, Journal of Biological Chemistry, and Journal of Pharmacology and Experimental Therapeutics. In 2012, Karen joined the editorial staff at WilliamsTown Communications, an editing firm that specializes in educational products for undergraduate- and graduate-level students. At WTC, Karen specializes in producing educational products related to the sciences and healthcare. In addition, Karen is board-certified for editing life sciences (BELS-certified).

A Note from the Authors

Thank you for purchasing our book! Worldwide, over forty million people suffer from Alzheimer's disease, and that number is expected to increase significantly within the next fifteen years. In the United States, over five million people have the disease, and that is expected to triple by the year 2050.

Despite these large numbers, you may feel alone. I (Laura) know that when I started caring for my father, who had early-onset Alzheimer's disease, I felt alone. Although my father has passed away, I am haunted by what he suffered and how difficult it was to care for him. However, now I know that there are people, resources, and organizations that can help others going through this same struggle.

We recognize that caregivers have emotional, physical, and financial challenges. We hope that the information in the Alzheimer's Roadmap series will ease some of your stress. The information included in this book can help you manage your loved one's finances and healthcare costs and understand the complicated world of government resources. In addition, we have included resources at the end of this book to provide additional information to help you through this process.

If you have any questions for us, feel free to post them on Laura Town's Amazon Author Central page or reach out to the authors via twitter: @laurawtown. We would appreciate it if you would take the time to review our book on Amazon, as our book's visibility on Amazon depends on reviews.

Additional Titles from Laura Town and Karen Hoffman

Alzheimer's Roadmap series:

Long-Term Care Insurance, Power of Attorney, Wealth Management, and Other First Steps

Dementia, Alzheimer's Disease Stages, Treatment Options, and Other Medical Considerations

Advance Directives, Durable Power of Attorney, Wills, and Other Legal Considerations

Paying for Healthcare and Other Financial Considerations

Home Safety Checklist Guide and Caregiver Resources for Medication Safety, Driving, and Wandering

Home Care, Long-term Care, Memory Care Units, and Other Living Arrangements

Caregiver Resources for Helping with Activities of Daily Living

Nutrition for Brain Health: Fighting Dementia

Caregiver Resources: From Independence to a Memory Care Unit

Coping with Dementia

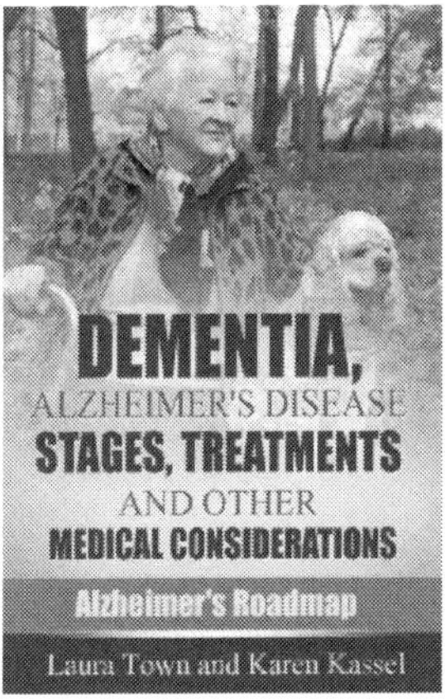

Know What to Expect

Dementia, Alzheimer's Disease Stages, Treatments, and Other Medical Considerations provides answers to the following questions and more:

- **What is Alzheimer's disease?** Learn what Alzheimer's disease is, including its characteristics, signs, and risk factors.
- **What can my loved one with Alzheimer's disease expect?** Read detailed descriptions of the stages of Alzheimer's disease, including what patients and caregivers can expect to see at each stage as the disease progresses.
- **What treatments are available?** A survey of prescription medications introduces you to the treatments available to help patients cope with the progression of the disease.
- **What about clinical trials?** Clinical trials are important to finding a cure for Alzheimer's disease, but this book describes the precautions for your loved one to consider before choosing to participate in them.
- **Is there audio for this book?** Yes, you can find the audiobook here: https://adbl.co/2SwzzlA.

Resources

Information about Alzheimer's Disease

Alzheimer's Association
225 N. Michigan Ave., Fl. 17
Chicago, IL 60601-7633
Phone: 800-272-3900
Fax: 866-699-1246
Email: info@alz.org
Website: http://www.alz.org

Alzheimer's Disease Education and Referral (ADEAR) Center
National Institute on Aging
Building 31, Room 5C27
31 Center Drive, MSC 2292
Bethesda, MD 20892
Phone: 800-438-4380
Email: adear@nia.nih.gov
Website: https://www.nia.nih.gov/health/alzheimers

Alzheimer's Foundation of America
322 Eighth Ave., 7th fl.
New York, NY 10001
Phone: 866-232-8484
Fax: 646-638-1546
Email: info@alzfdn.org
Website: www.alzfdn.org

Fisher Center for Alzheimer's Research Foundation
110 East 42nd Street, 16th Floor
New York, NY 10017
Phone: 1-800-ALZINFO (259-4636)
Fax: 1-212-915-1319
Email: info@alzinfo.org
Website: https://www.alzinfo.org/

National Institute on Aging
Website: https://www.nia.nih.gov/
Specific helpful websites:
https://www.nia.nih.gov/health/alzheimers
https://www.nia.nih.gov/health/end-of-life

Information about Hospice and Palliative Care

Mayo Clinic
200 First St. SW
Rochester, MN 55905
Phone: 507-284-2511
Website: http://www.mayoclinic.org/
Specific helpful website:
https://www.mayoclinic.org/tests-procedures/palliative-care/about/pac-20384637

National Hospice and Palliative Care Organization
1731 King Street
Alexandria, VA 22314
Phone: 703-837-1500
Fax: 703-837-1233
Website: http://www.nhpco.org/
Specific helpful websites:
http://www.nhpco.org/about/hospice-care

U.S. National Library of Medicine
8600 Rockville Pike
Bethesda, MD 20894
Phone: (888) FIND-NLM
Website: http://www.nlm.nih.gov/
Specific helpful website:
http://www.nlm.nih.gov/medlineplus/hospicecare.html

Information about Artificial Nutrition, Hydration, and Respiration

American Hospice Foundation
Website: http://americanhospice.org/
Specific helpful website:
http://americanhospice.org/caregiving/artificial-nutrition-and-hydration-at-the-end-of-life-beneficial-or-harmful/

Family Caregiver Alliance
101 Montgomery Street, Suite 2150
San Francisco, CA 94104
Phone: 1-(800)-445-8106
Website: https://www.caregiver.org/
Specific helpful website:
https://www.caregiver.org/advanced-illness-feeding-tubes-and-ventilators

Information about Grieving

Alzheimer's Association
225 N. Michigan Ave., Fl. 17
Chicago, IL 60601-7633
Phone: 800-272-3900
Fax: 866-699-1246
Email: info@alz.org
Website: http://www.alz.org
Specific helpful website:
https://www.alz.org/help-support/caregiving/caregiver-health/grief-loss-as-alzheimers-progresses

American Hospice Foundation
Website: http://americanhospice.org/
Specific helpful website:
http://americanhospice.org/working-through-grief/

Mayo Clinic
200 First St. SW
Rochester, MN 55905
Phone: 507-284-2511
Website: http://www.mayoclinic.org/
Specific helpful website:
http://www.mayoclinic.org/healthy-lifestyle/end-of-life/expert-answers/grieving-process/faq-20058274

Information about Funeral Services

Alzheimer's Association
225 N. Michigan Ave., Fl. 17
Chicago, IL 60601-7633
Phone: 800-272-3900
Fax: 866-699-1246
Email: info@alz.org
Website: http://www.alz.org
Specific helpful website:
https://www.alz.org/help-support/i-have-alz/plan-for-your-future/end_of_life_planning

Federal Trade Commission
600 Pennsylvania Avenue, NW
Washington, DC 20580
Phone: (202) 326-2222
Complaint form: https://www.ftccomplaintassistant.gov
Website: http://www.consumer.ftc.gov/
Specific helpful website:
http://www.consumer.ftc.gov/articles/0301-funeral-costs-and-pricing-checklist

Funeral Consumers Alliance
33 Patchen Road
South Burlington, VT 05403
Phone: 802-865-8300

Website: http://www.funerals.org/
Specific helpful website:
https://funerals.org/consumers/

Information about Estate Planning

Fisher Center for Alzheimer's Research Foundation
110 East 42nd Street, 16th Floor
New York, NY 10017
Phone: 1-800-ALZINFO (259-4636)
Fax: 1-212-915-1319
Email: info@alzinfo.org
Website: https://www.alzinfo.org/
Specific helpful website:
https://www.alzinfo.org/articles/estate-planning/

Internal Revenue Service
Website for contacting your local IRS office:
https://www.irs.gov/help/contact-your-local-irs-office
Website: http://www.irs.gov/
Specific helpful website:
https://www.irs.gov/businesses/small-businesses-self-employed/deceased-taxpayers-understanding-the-general-duties-as-an-estate-administrator

Social Security Administration
Office of Public Inquiries and Communications Support
1100 West High Rise
6401 Security Blvd.
Baltimore, MD 21235
Phone: 1-800-772-1213
Email form: https://secure.ssa.gov/emailus/
Website: http://www.ssa.gov/
Specific helpful website:
http://www.ssa.gov/planners/survivors/onyourown.html

Reference List

Abrahms, S. (2019). Preparing for the loss of a parent. Retrieved from https://www.aplaceformom.com/blog/10-24-14-prepare-for-loss/

Alzheimer's Association. (2017). Autopsy, brain and body donation and low-cost funeral and burial options. Retrieved from https://www.alz.org/media/greatermissouri/Autopsy_Brain_and_Body_donation_Low-cost_funeral_and_burial_options.pdf

Alzheimer's Association. (2019). End-of-life planning. Retrieved from https://www.alz.org/help-support/i-have-alz/plan-for-your-future/end_of_life_planning

Alzheimer's Association. (2019). Late-stage caregiving. Retrieved from https://www.alz.org/help-support/caregiving/stages-behaviors/late-stage

Alzheimer's Association. (2019). Grief and loss as Alzheimer's progresses. Retrieved from https://www.alz.org/help-support/caregiving/caregiver-health/grief-loss-as-alzheimers-progresses

Alzheimer Society of Canada. (2019). Comforting the person. Retrieved from https://alzheimer.ca/en/Home/Living-with-dementia/Caring-for-someone/End-of-life-care/Comforting

Alzheimer Society of Canada. (2016). Progression. Retrieved from https://alzheimer.ca/sites/default/files/files/national/progression-series/progression_end-of-life.pdf

Alzheimer's Society. (n.d.). End of life care. Retrieved from https://www.alzheimers.org.uk/get-support/help-dementia-care/end-life-care

American Psychological Association. (2011). Grief: Coping with the loss of your loved one. Retrieved from http://www.apa.org/helpcenter/grief.aspx

Arenella, C. (n.d.) Artificial nutrition and hydration at the end of life: Beneficial or harmful? Retrieved from http://americanhospice.org/caregiving/artificial-nutrition-and-hydration-at-the-end-of-life-beneficial-or-harmful/

Center for Hospice Care. (2018). Know the difference: Hospice vs. palliative care. Retrieved from https://www.hospicesect.org/hospice-and-palliative-care

Creagana, E. T. (2017). Is it possible to grieve the death of a loved one without crying? Retrieved from https://www.mayoclinic.org/healthy-lifestyle/end-of-life/expert-answers/grieving-process/faq-20058274

Creagan, E. T. (2018). Dealing with grief: Confronting painful emotions. Retrieved from http://www.mayoclinic.org/healthy-living/end-of-life/in-depth/grief/art-20047261?pg=2

Crossroads Hospice & Palliative Care. (2019). Blood pressure before death. Retrieved from https://www.crossroadshospice.com/hospice-caregiver-support/end-of-life-signs/blood-pressure/

Crossroads Hospice & Palliative Care. (2019). Breathing patterns before death. Retrieved from https://www.crossroadshospice.com/hospice-caregiver-support/end-of-life-signs/breathing-patterns/

Crossroads Hospice & Palliative Care. (2019). Preparing for the death of a parent. Retrieved from https://www.crossroadshospice.com/hospice-caregiver-support/end-of-life-signs/death-of-a-parent/

Crossroads Hospice & Palliative Care. (2019). Signs of dying in the elderly with dementia. Retrieved from https://www.crossroadshospice.com/hospice-caregiver-support/end-of-life-signs/dementia/

Family Caregiver Alliance. (2013). Advanced illness: Feeding tubes and ventilators. Retrieved from https://www.caregiver.org/advanced-illness-feeding-tubes-and-ventilators

FamilyDoctor.org. (2018). Artificial hydration and nutrition. Retrieved from https://familydoctor.org/artificial-hydration-and-nutrition/

Federal Trade Commission. (2012). Funeral costs and pricing checklist. Retrieved from https://www.consumer.ftc.gov/articles/0301-funeral-costs-and-pricing-checklist

Federal Trade Commission. (2012). Types of funerals. Retrieved from https://www.consumer.ftc.gov/articles/0302-types-funerals

Financial Samurai. (2016). Preparing for death: A checklist for the inevitable. Retrieved from https://www.financialsamurai.com/preparing-for-death-a-checklist-for-the-inevitable/

Fisher Center for Alzheimer's Research Foundation. (2019). Clinical stages of Alzheimer's. Retrieved from https://www.alzinfo.org/understand-alzheimers/clinical-stages-of-alzheimers/

Fisher Center for Alzheimer's Research Foundation. (2019). Estate planning. Retrieved from https://www.alzinfo.org/articles/estate-planning/

Fitzgerald, H. (n.d.) Alzheimer's disease and grieving caregivers. Retrieved from http://americanhospice.org/caregiving/alzheimers-disease-and-grieving-caregivers/

Get Palliative Care. (2019). Disease types and palliative care. Retrieved from https://getpalliativecare.org/whatis/disease-types/

Heerema, E. (2018). Signs of infection in dementia and Alzheimer's. Retrieved from https://www.verywellhealth.com/how-do-infections-affect-people-with-dementia-98860

Internal Revenue Service. (2018). Deceased taxpayers – Understanding the general duties as an estate administrator. Retrieved from http://www.irs.gov/Businesses/Small-Businesses-&-Self-Employed/Deceased-Taxpayers-Understanding-the-General-Duties-as-an-Estate-Administrator

Irving, S. (2019). How to get a death certificate. Retrieved from https://www.nolo.com/legal-encyclopedia/how-get-death-certificate.html

Kirk, S. (2010). Artificial nutrition and hydration. Retrieved from http://www.azbioethicsnetwork.org/resources/encyclopedia/artificial-nutrition-and-hydration

Kotterman, J. D. S. (2018). What I wished I knew before my mother's Alzheimer's death. Retrieved from https://www.beingpatient.com/alzheimers-death/

Mayo Clinic. (2017). Heart failure. Retrieved from https://www.mayoclinic.org/diseases-conditions/heart-failure/symptoms-causes/syc-20373142

Mayo Clinic. (2017). Palliative care. Retrieved from https://www.mayoclinic.org/tests-procedures/palliative-care/about/pac-20384637

Memorial Sloan Kettering Cancer Center. (2018). Toward the end of life: What you and your family can expect. Retrieved from https://www.mskcc.org/cancer-care/patient-education/towards-end-life

MyHealth.Alberta.ca. (2019). Symptom management – Bowel & bladder. Retrieved from https://myhealth.alberta.ca/palliative-care/resources/symptom-management/bowel-and-bladder-problems

National Hospice and Palliative Care Organization. (2019). Hospice care. Retrieved from http://www.nhpco.org/about/hospice-care

National Hospice and Palliative Care Organization. (n.d.). Hospice eligibility requirements. Retrieved from https://www.nhpco.org/hospice-eligibility-requirements

National Institute on Aging. (n.d.). Alzheimer's disease & related dementias. Retrieved from https://www.nia.nih.gov/health/alzheimers

National Institute on Aging. (n.d.). End of life. Retrieved from https://www.nia.nih.gov/health/end-of-life

National Institute on Aging. (2017). What are palliative care and hospice care? Retrieved from https://www.nia.nih.gov/health/what-are-palliative-care-and-hospice-care

National Institute on Aging. (2018). Pain: You can get help. Retrieved from https://www.nia.nih.gov/health/pain-you-can-get-help

National Institute on Aging. (2019). Alzheimer's Disease Research Centers. Retrieved from https://www.nia.nih.gov/health/alzheimers-disease-research-centers#kansas

National Pressure Ulcer Advisory Panel. (2016). NPUAP Pressure injury stages. Retrieved from https://www.npuap.org/resources/educational-and-clinical-resources/npuap-pressure-injury-stages/

Pathways. (2019). How do you become eligible for hospice? Retrieved from https://www.pathwayshealth.org/hospice-topics/become-eligible-hospice/

Prince William County Virginia Clerk of Circuit Court. (n.d.) Probate frequently asked questions. Retrieved from http://www.pwcgov.org/government/courts/circuit/Pages/Probate-Frequently-Asked-Questions.aspx#faq19

Salamat, S., & Fruehling, J. (2019). How brain autopsies are helping further dementia research. Retrieved from https://www.adrc.wisc.edu/dementia-matters/how-brain-autopsies-are-helping-further-dementia-research

Smith, M., Robinson, L., & Segal, J. (2019). Coping with grief and loss. Retrieved from http://www.helpguide.org/articles/grief-loss/coping-with-grief-and-loss.htm

Social Security Administration. (2019). Benefits planner: Survivors. Retrieved from http://www.ssa.gov/planners/survivors/onyourown.html

Stevenson, S. (2019). How to recognize the signs of anticipatory grief. Retrieved from https://www.aplaceformom.com/blog/1-27-15-signs-of-anticipatory-grief/

U.S. National Library of Medicine: Medline Plus. (2018). Hospice care. Retrieved from https://medlineplus.gov/hospicecare.html

U.S. National Library of Medicine: Medline Plus. (2019). What is palliative care? Retrieved from https://medlineplus.gov/ency/patientinstructions/000536.htm

Wegerer, J. (2017). The connection between UTIs and dementia. Retrieved from https://www.alzheimers.net/2014-04-03/connection-between-utis-and-dementia/

Continue reading to see a selection from another Omega Press title, available now on Amazon.

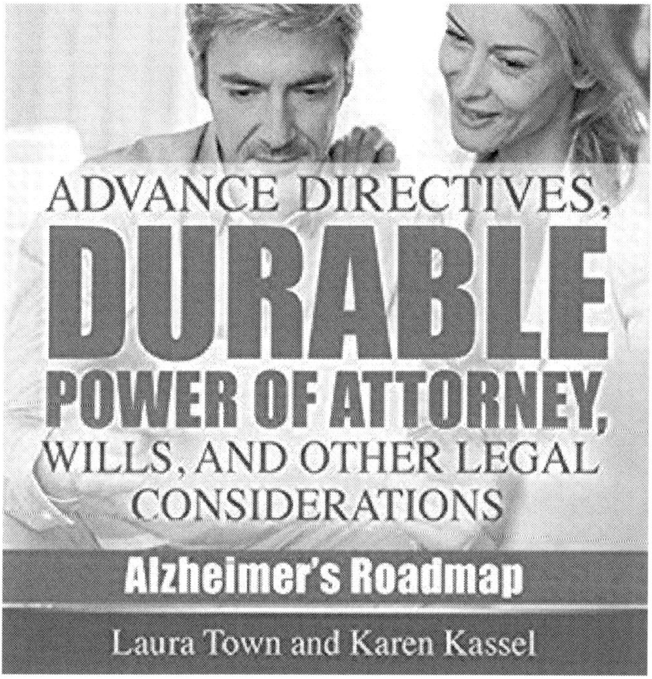

Legal Documents for Healthcare

Your loved one's need for good healthcare will grow as they progress through Alzheimer's disease. However, at some point in the course of the disease, your loved one will be unable to make their own healthcare choices, either because they cannot understand their medical choices, they cannot rationally make a decision, or they are unable to communicate their wishes. Therefore, having legal documents related to their healthcare wishes is vital to them receiving the care they would have chosen for themselves. Legal documents related to healthcare include a durable power of attorney for healthcare, living will, and other advance directives.

Durable Power of Attorney for Healthcare

A durable power of attorney for healthcare is created to name a single individual or group of individuals who will be allowed to make healthcare decisions for your loved one. A durable power of attorney for healthcare is called "durable" because it is active both before and after the principal is declared mentally incompetent. Choosing a good healthcare agent is one of the most important legal decisions your loved one will make. The following checklists include important aspects to consider when creating a durable power of attorney for healthcare.

Checklist: Basics about a durable power of attorney for healthcare

- ☐ The durable power of attorney for healthcare document may also be called a healthcare power of attorney, medical power of attorney, appointment of a healthcare agent, or healthcare proxy.
- ☐ The individual creating the durable power of attorney for healthcare is called the *principal.* In this book, your loved one with Alzheimer's disease is assumed to be the principal.
- ☐ The individual named to make healthcare decisions for the principal is called the *healthcare agent.* They may also be called a surrogate, attorney-in-fact, healthcare representative, or healthcare proxy.
- ☐ The healthcare agent is only allowed to make medical decisions, not financial decisions, for your loved one.
- ☐ The durable power of attorney for healthcare is valid for both temporary (e.g., after an accident) and permanent (e.g., late-stage Alzheimer's disease) incapacitation.
- ☐ Although the durable power of attorney for healthcare is valid as soon as it is signed, physicians usually do not take advice from the healthcare agent as long as your loved one is capable of making decisions.

- ☐ The durable power of attorney for healthcare can be revoked or changed at any time, as long as your loved one is still legally competent.
- ☐ Your loved one should include a HIPAA release in the durable power of attorney for healthcare so the healthcare agent can access your loved one's medical records.
- ☐ A major benefit to having a healthcare agent compared to only a living will is that the healthcare agent can make all healthcare decisions in real time based on current information; the living will is designed for a limited number of hypothetical situations.
- ☐ If your loved one becomes incapacitated and does not have a healthcare agent, he or she will either be appointed a healthcare proxy by a physician (a short-term solution) or will need to have a guardian appointed by the court (a long-term solution).

Checklist: Responsibilities of the principal

- ☐ Determine if there are any state laws restricting the choice of healthcare agent. For example, does the healthcare agent have to be a resident of the same state as your loved one?
- ☐ Choose a healthcare agent based on desired characteristics of a healthcare agent. Make sure the chosen agent is willing to accept this responsibility. Some states require that only one healthcare agent has power at a time, but some allow multiple agents.

- ☐ If more than one healthcare agent is chosen to act at the same time, all agents must be present and agree on medical actions before medical personnel will act on the decisions. This makes it complicated for physicians to act, especially if the agents do not agree.
- ☐ Choose an alternative healthcare agent if the original healthcare agent is unavailable or is unwilling to serve.
- ☐ Stipulate any restrictions on the healthcare agent, such as when the agent can make decisions (e.g., after diagnosis of a terminal illness, when the principal is permanently unconscious, etc.).
- ☐ Name any individuals who should *not* have any role in making healthcare decisions. This may be an estranged family member or in-laws.
- ☐ Create and sign the durable power of attorney for healthcare document. If your loved one spends significant time in more than one state, a durable power of attorney for healthcare document should be created for each state.
- ☐ Distribute copies of the durable power of attorney for healthcare to regular healthcare providers, the local hospital, the healthcare agent and alternative healthcare agent, and close family members.
- ☐ Keep a copy of the durable power of attorney document in an easily accessible place at home, and tell the healthcare agent and close family members where to find the document.

- ☐ Discuss responsibilities of the healthcare agent and any advance directives with the chosen agent(s).
- ☐ Discuss with the healthcare agent any values and beliefs that would affect healthcare decisions. Examples are religious beliefs that would dictate refusal of medical treatments, aspects that give your loved one's life meaning (family, career, independence, etc.), concerns about death or dying, and financial concerns.
- ☐ Tell family members whom the chosen healthcare agent is and why.
- ☐ If one healthcare agent become unwilling or unable to serve, or if your loved one wishes to revoke the agent's power, your loved one will need to create a new document and destroy all old documents.

Checklist: Characteristics of a good healthcare agent

- ☐ Meets the state's legal requirements for healthcare agent, including being over age 18.
- ☐ Will likely be available until your loved one's death (i.e., not someone who is close to death or has a terminal illness).
- ☐ Has a close, amicable relationship with your loved one; someone your loved one trusts with his or her life.
- ☐ Willing to take on the role of healthcare agent.

- ☐ Understands the significance of the healthcare agent role.
- ☐ Willing to discuss sensitive issues with your loved one.
- ☐ Shares your loved one's views and values regarding life, death, and medical treatments.
- ☐ Willing to follow all the stipulations in the living will, even if the agent does not agree with the stipulations.
- ☐ Willing to stand firm in the face of adversity if others do not agree with your loved one's wishes.
- ☐ Lives in close proximity to your loved one and is available to attend doctor's appointments or could travel to be close by if needed.
- ☐ Flexible and able to stay calm under pressure.
- ☐ Level-headed and mature.
- ☐ Not afraid to ask questions of care providers.
- ☐ Not easily intimidated or overwhelmed by medical jargon or information.
- ☐ Not someone your loved one picks out of guilt or obligation.
- ☐ Not someone who is your loved one's healthcare provider, a relative of a healthcare provider, an employee at a business or government agency that finances your loved one's healthcare, or anyone else who may have a conflict of interest.

- ☐ Common choices include a spouse, life partner, adult child, sibling, or trusted friend.

Checklist: Responsibilities of a healthcare agent

Before making healthcare decisions:

- ☐ Discuss healthcare preferences with your loved one, including wishes for life-sustaining treatments. This should include preferences listed in your loved one's living will.
- ☐ Understand your loved one's current medications, including dosing and scheduling, as well as any allergies.
- ☐ Make sure physicians and other healthcare personnel as well as close family members have the most recent copies of all healthcare-related legal documents, such as power of attorney, living will, and advance directives.
- ☐ Carry a copy of the durable power of attorney for healthcare with you to show to facilities in case they have misplaced their copy.
- ☐ Ensure that the power of attorney document will be accepted by clinics, hospitals, and healthcare providers.
- ☐ Make sure the medical staff understands that you are the healthcare agent.

Making decisions:

- ☐ Receive and understand information about your loved one's medical condition, including prognosis with and without treatment. Stay informed as your loved one's medical condition changes.

- ☐ Be present for support and consultation during medical tests and procedures.
- ☐ Access your loved one's medical records; because of HIPAA laws, the healthcare agent must present the durable power of attorney for healthcare document in order to be granted access to medical records.
- ☐ Discuss healthcare options with the medical team; understand the pros and cons of different treatment options. Write down information as needed.
- ☐ Write down questions to ask the physician, and ask them at the next opportunity. Prioritize more important questions first.
- ☐ Seek second opinions as needed.
- ☐ Get support from medical staff for decisions, including physicians, nurses, social workers, chaplains, and ethics committee members.
- ☐ Make healthcare decisions for your loved one; decisions should be similar to choices your loved one would make and in your loved one's best interest.
- ☐ After decisions have been made, pass the decisions on to healthcare workers and caregivers.
- ☐ Sign consent forms for medical procedures.

Types of decisions:

- ☐ Choose your loved one's physicians and other healthcare providers.
- ☐ Choose care facilities for your loved one.
- ☐ Approve a transfer of care between facilities or between physicians.
- ☐ Approve medical treatments that your loved one will receive, including but not limited to medications, therapy, and surgery.
- ☐ Withhold or withdraw medical treatments according to the living will or your loved one's religious or cultural views, such as withholding artificial nutrition and hydration or blood transfusions.
- ☐ Authorize or refuse participation in medical research; can also authorize the experimental treatments be stopped.
- ☐ Approve or revoke DNR or DNI (Do Not Intubate) orders after discussing the pros and cons with a physician.
- ☐ Choose whether your loved one will die at home or in a healthcare facility.
- ☐ Decide when to start or stop providing only palliative care, comfort care, or hospice care.
- ☐ Give consent for organ donation and autopsy; your loved one's preference for this may be in the living will.

Printed in Great Britain
by Amazon

48037408R00061